1992 JOINT COMMISSION

AMAHC

Accreditation Manual for Ambulatory Health Care
Volume I Standards

Celebrating • 40 Years • of • Quality • Improvement

JOINT COMMISSION MISSION

The mission of the Joint Commission on Accreditation of Healthcare Organizations is to improve the quality of health care provided to the public. The Joint Commission develops standards of quality in collaboration with health professionals and others and stimulates health care organizations to meet or exceed the standards through accreditation and the teaching of quality improvement concepts.

Printed in the United States of America
ISBN: 0-86688-278-2
Copyright © 1992 by the Joint Commission on Accreditation of Healthcare Organizations

Requests for permission to make copies of any part of this work should be mailed to Permissions Editor, Department of Publications, Joint Commission on Accreditation of Healthcare Organizations, One Renaissance Boulevard, Oakbrook Terrace, IL 60181.

Address orders to Customer Service Center, Joint Commission on Accreditation of Healthcare Organizations, One Renaissance Boulevard, Oakbrook Terrace, IL 60181.

Questions about standards and/or guidelines should be referred to Department of Standards, Joint Commission on Accreditation of Healthcare Organizations, One Renaissance Boulevard, Oakbrook Terrace, IL 60181.

Questions about the use of these standards in the survey process should be referred to Long Term Care Accreditation Services, Joint Commission on Accreditation of Healthcare Organizations, One Renaissance Boulevard, Oakbrook Terrace, IL 60181.

Address editorial correspondence to Department of Publications, Joint Commission on Accreditation of Healthcare Organizations, One Renaissance Boulevard, Oakbrook Terrace, IL 60181.

FOREWORD

The 1992 *Accreditation Manual for Ambulatory Health Care (AMAHC)* marks the beginning of a transition to standards intended to encourage the application of continuous quality improvement (CQI) principles in ambulatory health care organizations. This transition is one of the three major initiatives that make up the Joint Commission's Agenda for Change. The remaining initiatives involve the development and use of performance measures (indicators) and of an indicator data base designed to support ongoing measurement, monitoring, and improvement of facility performance and a major redesign of the accreditation survey process to focus primary attention on actual organizational performance.

The new *AMAHC* begins a standards transition that is expected to continue at least through the 1996 edition. A "Quality Assessment and Improvement" chapter, which replaces the former "Quality Assurance" chapter, includes new standards for monitoring and evaluation that are intended to facilitate the shift within organizations from quality assurance to quality improvement. The changes are also designed to support organizations in adopting more modern approaches to quality assessment.

Revisions in other chapters respond to a growing interest in addressing the needs of the terminally ill patient. In addition, standards relating to summary list requirements have been revised to clarify both the requirement and its use in promoting continuity of care.

The 1992 *AMAHC* appears in a two-volume format. Volume I contains the standards and will be familiar to you as the biennial *Ambulatory Health Care Standards Manual*. Volume II contains the scoring guidelines for the standards. New scoring guidelines for administration, educational activities, governing body, research activities, rights and responsibilities of patients, and teaching and publication activities are included.

As in the past, we invite your comments and suggestions regarding this *Manual*. In particular, we invite your thoughts about the new directions reflected by the Agenda for Change. The envisioned transition has been carefully structured to afford ample opportunity for input from, and discussion with, accredited organizations. We count on your participation in framing the expectations to be set forth in future editions of this *Manual*.

Dennis S. O'Leary, MD
President

CONTENTS

USING THE MANUAL

Volume I of the *Accreditation Manual for Ambulatory Health Care* is designed for use in self-assessment by ambulatory care organizations and is the basis for the survey report form, which Joint Commission surveyors use to record their on-site survey findings. The accreditation report sent to the organization directly quotes standards, permitting organization personnel to consult specific provisions of this *Manual* in carrying out postsurvey recommendations.

All chapters of this *Manual* are in outline format, which is intended to enhance readability, to clarify the intent of each standard and required characteristic, and to facilitate use of this *Manual* as a self-assessment guide. The numbering system used for the standards makes it easy to reference appropriate chapters. Each standard and required characteristic is given a two-letter code standing for the title of the chapter in which it appears; it is then numbered according to order of appearance within the chapter.

The standards and required characteristics that are most important to the accreditation decision process (key factors) are highlighted throughout this *Manual*. Although all standards have important implications for the delivery of high quality health care, those identified with an asterisk are central to the accreditation decision. The asterisks are intended to assist ambulatory care organizations in assessing their compliance with the key requirements.

The rating scale, which is used by surveyors to assess and report levels of compliance with standards, contains six rankings—the numbers 1 through 5 and NA (not applicable). This scale may also be used by organization staff in self-assessment. An explanation of the scale follows:

1 **Substantial compliance,** indicating that the organization consistently meets all major provisions of the standard or required characteristic.

2 **Significant compliance,** indicating that the organization meets most provisions of the standard or required characteristic.

3 **Partial compliance,** indicating that the organization meets some provisions of the standard or required characteristic.

4 **Minimal compliance,** indicating that the organization meets few provisions of the standard or required characteristic.

5 **Noncompliance,** indicating that the organization fails to meet the provisions of the standard or required characteristic.

NA **Not applicable,** indicating that the standard or required characteristic does not apply to the organization.

Space is provided at the end of each chapter for organization staff conducting a self-assessment to record comments and note actions to be taken to bring the organization into compliance with specific standards and required characteristics.

Self-assessments are a valuable management aid because they provide staff with information about the quality of services provided in their organization. Each organization should determine how it will use this *Manual* as a self-assessment tool. For example, someone could be assigned to conduct an evaluation of all the services, or the person responsible for each service could conduct an evaluation of that service. Whatever method is used, the important point is that self-assessments should be done routinely according to a schedule established by the organization. Management and staff can use the results of self-assessments to plan corrective actions for areas that need improvement and to help ensure compliance with standards.

As part of their self-evaluation activities, organization staff members are strongly encouraged to read *Joint Commission Perspectives,* the official bimonthly newsletter of the Joint Commission. All changes in standards and in survey policies and procedures are reported promptly in this newsletter.

GENERAL ADMINISTRATIVE POLICIES AND PROCEDURES

SURVEY ELIGIBILITY CRITERIA

Any ambulatory health care organization or program may apply for a Joint Commission accreditation survey if the following eligibility requirements are met:

- The organization or program is located within the United States or one of its territories or possessions or is a Department of Defense medical treatment facility/program.
- The organization or program is a formally organized and legally constituted entity that primarily provides ambulatory health care services, or is a subunit that primarily provides such services within a formally organized and legally constituted entity that is not necessarily health care related.
- The organization or program provides the direct services of physicians.
- The organization or program shares the facilities, equipment, business management, and records involved in patient care among the members of the organization.
- The organization or program is in compliance with applicable federal, state, and local law and regulation, including any requirements for licensure.
- The organization or program is currently in operation and actively caring for patients. When the organization or program has been in operation for less than six months, the accreditation award automatically includes a follow-up visit so that the organization's or program's record of performance can be evaluated.
- The organization or program completes and returns an Application for Survey with the nonrefundable processing fee.
- The organization or program completes presurvey materials as directed.
- The organization or program operates without restriction by reason of sex, race, creed, or national origin.

With the exceptions of the offices of physicians in solo practice, any organization or program that meets the eligibility criteria may apply for a Joint Commission accreditation survey. The accreditation program is intended primarily for the following types of organizations and programs:

- Ambulatory care clinics;
- Ambulatory surgery centers;
- College or university health programs;
- Community health centers;
- Single and multispecialty group practices;
- Armed Services programs;
- Cardiac catheterization centers;
- Native American health service centers;
- Primary care centers;
- Urgent/emergency care centers;
- Physical rehabilitation centers;

- Staff and group model HMOs;
- Correctional health programs;
- Endoscopy centers;
- Infusion therapy centers;
- Corporate and occupational health programs; and
- Diagnostic imaging centers.

Organizations and programs are considered for survey on an individual basis. The Joint Commission determines whether the standards can be applied appropriately to a given applicant. If the standards cannot be applied, a survey will not be conducted. The organization or program is informed of the reason for such a decision, and the application fee is refunded.

CONFIDENTIALITY AND DISCLOSURE

Confidentiality
The Joint Commission treats as confidential the following information that is received or developed during the accreditation process:

- Information obtained from an organization before, during, and/or following the accreditation survey;
- All materials that may contribute to the accreditation decision (for example, surveyor report forms);
- Standards compliance recommendations; and
- Written staff analyses and Accreditation Committee minutes and agenda materials.

This policy applies to all ambulatory health care organizations that have an accreditation history, except as provided below or as otherwise provided by law or as authorized by responsible officials of the organization.

Disclosure
A. Information Subject to Public Release
The Joint Commission, upon request, will publicly release the following information:

- Current accreditation status of an ambulatory health care organization;
- Organization accreditation history;
- The date(s) of a scheduled survey after an organization has been notified;
- The status of an organization in the accreditation decision process;
- Applicable standards under which an accreditation survey was conducted;
- Organizational and operational components included in the accreditation survey;
- The applicable standards areas involved in a Joint Commission complaint investigation;
- For a tailored survey, the organizational component(s) that contributed to a decision of conditional accreditation or denial of accreditation; and
- Whether, at the time an organization withdrew from accreditation, there were any type I recommendations for which the Joint Commission had no or insufficient evidence of resolution.

B. Aggregate Data
The Joint Commission reserves the prerogative to publish, or otherwise release publicly, aggregate standards compliance or related data that do not identify individual organizations.

C. Information Subject to Release to Responsible Government Agencies*

The Joint Commission provides to responsible federal, state, or local government agencies the information specified below under the following circumstances:

- When a serious situation that may jeopardize the safety of patients or the public is identified in an organization by a Joint Commission surveyor, and the chief executive officer has been advised of the situation, local, state, and federal authorities having jurisdiction over the organization will immediately be notified by the Joint Commission by telephone and in writing.

- When an organization is certified for participation in the Medicare program as a consequence of accreditation or is licensed on the basis of its accreditation (as provided in statute or regulation) and becomes conditionally accredited or not accredited, relevant Joint Commission accreditation survey information will be provided to the Administrator of the Health Care Financing Administration and, as appropriate, to the applicable state licensure agency. The information provided is to be limited to the following:

  — All type I recommendations;

  — A brief summary indicating the general standards areas in which the organization is in at least significant compliance and the general areas of noncompliance;

  — A statement, if any, provided by the organization regarding the validity of the Joint Commission survey findings; and

  — For conditionally accredited organizations, a copy of the approved plan of correction and subsequently the results of the plan-of-correction follow-up survey.

D. Policy Oversight and Special Information Requests

The Executive Committee of the Board of Commissioners shall provide oversight of execution of this policy and shall determine the handling of official specific information requests (for example, from government agencies).

HOW TO APPLY FOR SURVEY

Organizations that wish to be accredited by the Joint Commission should begin by sending a request for an Application for Survey to the following address:

> Joint Commission on Accreditation of Healthcare Organizations
> Scheduling Department—Application Requests
> One Renaissance Boulevard
> Oakbrook Terrace, Illinois 60181

The Joint Commission sends the organization one application for completion. In submitting its application, the organization authorizes the Joint Commission to obtain official records and reports of public or publicly recognized licensing, examining, reviewing, or planning bodies. The organization also has an obligation to furnish such documents in its possession to the Joint Commission, if requested

Section 92, PL 96-499, the Omnibus Reconciliation Act of 1980, requires that Medicare providers include, in all their contracts for services costing $10,000 or more in any 12-month period, a clause allowing the Secretary of the U.S. Department of Health and Human Services (DHHS), the U.S. Comptroller General, or their representatives to examine the contract and the contractor's books and records. The Joint Commission herein stipulates that if its charges to any such organization amount to $10,000 or more in any 12-month period, the contract or any agreement on which such charges are based and any of the Joint Commission's books, documents, and records that may be necessary to verify the extent and nature of Joint Commission costs will be available to the Secretary of DHHS, the Comptroller General, or any of their duly authorized representatives for four years after the survey. The same conditions will apply to any subcontracts the Joint Commission has with related organizations if the payments under such contracts amount to $10,000 or more in any 12-month period.

to do so. The completed application should be returned to the Joint Commission. The organization should retain a copy of the application for its records. The Application for Survey, when accepted by the Joint Commission as reflected by notification to the organization of the scheduling of a survey, is the primary document establishing the terms of the relationship between the organization and the Joint Commission.

SURVEY FEES

Survey fees are related to the cost of maintaining Joint Commission operations and ordinarily are determined annually. Survey fees include a fixed base fee and an additional variable charge, which is related to the type and volume of services provided by the applicant organization. For more information on how survey fees are calculated, contact the Department of Planning and Financial Affairs at the Joint Commission corporate office.

When an organization is scheduled for survey, the Joint Commission sends an invoice and asks the organization to pay the fees in accordance with the terms specified. Organizations are charged at the fee rate in effect at the time of survey. For an initial survey (that is, an organization's first survey or its first survey after two or more years without Joint Commission accreditation), an organization must send a nonrefundable processing fee with the Application for Survey; this payment is credited toward the organization's total fee.

The Joint Commission offers two payment options. The organization can either pay the full survey fee when billed or spread the payments over a 3½-month period. Under the second option, an organization must pay half of the full survey fee at the time of billing (generally about four weeks before the date of the survey) and must pay the other half no later than 60 days after the date of the survey.

An organization that has not paid its survey fee in full prior to issuance of the accreditation decision and report will have 60 days from receipt of the report to remit the outstanding balance. Failure to provide timely payment may result in termination of accreditation. Organizations having significant standards compliance problems, as reflected by either a conditional accreditation decision or a decision to deny accreditation, are notified as soon as possible, whether or not payment has been received.

SURVEYS AND SCHEDULES

Accreditation surveys are conducted by Joint Commission surveyors. The number of days required for a survey and the composition of the survey team are based on information provided in the completed Application for Survey. If such information is discovered during the survey to have been inaccurate and supplied in error, any award of accreditation may be delayed, and the organization will be responsible to pay compensation for any unnecessary expenses incurred by the Joint Commission as a result. An organization may request a longer survey than that determined by the Joint Commission. A fee will be charged for the additional time. Such a request should be sent to the director of the Scheduling Department.

If, after mailing the application form and before the survey, the organization undergoes a change that renders inaccurate any information entered in the Application for Survey, the organization must notify the Scheduling Department immediately. Changes that must be reported include a change in ownership, a significant increase or decrease in the volume of services, the addition of a new type of health service, or the deletion of an existing service. If a survey team arrives at the organization and discovers that a change was not reported, the Joint Commission may survey, at a later date, any unreported services for which it has standards. Accreditation may not be granted if all services provided have not been surveyed.

The Joint Commission schedules a survey to renew an organization's accreditation near the end of the three-year accreditation cycle. This is referred to as the organization's triennial survey. Triennial surveys are ordinarily conducted no sooner than the month preceding an organization's survey anniversary date, unless otherwise authorized by the organization, and ordinarily no later than 60 days after the due date. The organization is notified of the survey dates a minimum of four weeks before the survey.

To minimize the impact of a survey on an organization's scheduled activities, the Joint Commission attempts to honor written requests that identify specific events and dates during which an organization prefers not to be surveyed. There may be circumstances, however, that prevent the Joint Commission from honoring such requests. The Joint Commission must receive these requests no later than four months before an organization's survey anniversary date. When possible, this request should be returned with the completed application. Failure by the organization to permit the accomplishment of a scheduled survey may be viewed by the Joint Commission as constituting an immediate withdrawal from the accreditation program.

SURVEY POSTPONEMENTS AND DELAYS

To keep survey fees to a minimum, the Joint Commission attempts to schedule surveys systematically and efficiently, so organizations are asked to accept scheduled survey dates. Nevertheless, the Joint Commission does provide for the postponement or delay of surveys. A postponement is a request for change after a survey has been scheduled. A delay is a request to change the survey due date before a triennial survey is scheduled. Request for a postponement or delay should be directed to the Joint Commission's Scheduling Department. Ordinarily, the Joint Commission will not postpone or delay a survey for more than six months.

Scheduled surveys may be postponed when one or more of the following events have happened:

- A natural disaster or other major unforeseen event has occurred and has totally or substantially disrupted operations;

- The organization is involved in a major strike, has ceased admitting patients, and is transferring patients to other facilities; or

- Patients or the organization or both are being moved to another building during the scheduled survey.

It should be noted that, under the circumstances noted above, the Joint Commission reserves the right to conduct an on-site survey if the organization continues to provide patient care services. Scheduled surveys also may be postponed when the Joint Commission has provided less than four weeks advance notice in writing or by telephone of the survey date(s).

A request for a survey delay may be granted if the delay requested is at most 60 days from the organization's due date and if the Joint Commission can accommodate the request without incurring direct expenses of $500 or more. A delay may also be granted to facilitate the sequential survey of organizations that are part of a multifacility system.

An organization that does not meet any of the criteria described in the previous two paragraphs still may be allowed to postpone or delay its survey if it pays a fee to defray costs. However, the Joint Commission reserves the right to deny any request for a postponement or delay, regardless of the organization's willingness to pay the fee.

If a survey is not scheduled within one year of the Joint Commission's receipt of the Application for Survey, the application is voided and the Joint Commission requires the submission of a new one to ensure that application information is up-to-date. For initial surveys only, a new nonrefundable processing fee is also required.

TAILORED SURVEYS

The Joint Commission has standards manuals for, and conducts surveys of, (1) hospitals, (2) non–hospital-based psychiatric and substance abuse organizations, including community mental health centers, and services for persons with mental retardation or other developmental disabilities, (3) long term care organizations, (4) home care organizations, and (5) ambulatory health care organizations. When an organization provides more than one of these categories of services, the Joint Commission will tailor its survey process to reflect the particular services offered by the organization. During the survey, the Joint Commission evaluates all health care services provided by the organization with the objective of a single accreditation decision and a single survey report.

In tailoring the survey process to the nature and needs of an organization, the Joint Commission uses the standards specifically related to each of the services provided by the organization. Before a tailored survey is conducted, the organization receives a copy of each of the standards manuals to be used in the survey. The Joint Commission determines which manuals are applicable based on the information provided in the Application for Survey.

The scope of a tailored survey is based on the scope of services provided by the organization that submits an application for survey. In complex organizations, the parent organization and/or its subcomponents will determine the identity of the applicant organization. With respect to the applicant organization, the scope of the tailored survey will include all services for which the Joint Commission has applicable standards that the organization represents itself as providing to the public and/or are owned or controlled by the organization and functionally integrated with it. Control will most commonly be evidenced by retention of budget approval authority by the organization's governing body and/or, where a separate governing body for the service exists, by substantial duplication (greater than 50%) of its membership with the membership of the organization's governing body. Organization representations as to the services that it provides will be assessed by examining organization letterhead, brochures that are used to inform the public of its services, and other available advertising media. When the applicant organization is not the parent organization, the parent organization may request the survey of other services that are under the aegis of the parent organization, either independently or in conjunction with the survey of the applicant organization, provided that the services are functionally integrated.

MODIFIED SURVEY PROCESS

The Joint Commission offers the option of a modified survey process to multifacility systems that own or lease at least two organizations. This option includes three components: a corporate orientation, consecutive survey of corporate-owned organizations, and a corporate summation. The orientation session provides an opportunity for corporate staff to orient the survey team to the structure and practices of the system. The survey team will also survey all centralized corporate services, documentation, and policies and procedures applicable to Joint Commission standards. After the last organization of a system is surveyed, the survey team holds a summation for the system's corporate office staff. The corporate orientation and corporate summation are charged at a fixed rate.

ACCREDITATION SURVEY PROCEDURES

The purpose of a Joint Commission accreditation survey is to assess the extent of an organization's compliance with applicable Joint Commission standards. Compliance is assessed through one or more of the following means:

* Documentation of compliance provided by organization personnel;

- Verbal information concerning the implementation of standards, or examples of their implementation, that will enable a judgment of compliance to be made; and
- On-site observations by Joint Commission surveyors.

These all assume good faith and frank participation by the organization in the survey process. Failure to so participate can be grounds for a decision to deny accreditation.

An organization must be prepared to provide evidence of its compliance with each standard that is applicable to its operations. To be accredited, an organization must demonstrate that it is in substantial compliance with the standards overall, not necessarily with each applicable standard.

In the event that a Joint Commission surveyor finds that some aspect of organization operations adversely affects patient health and safety, such findings may be considered for accreditation purposes even if the standards do not specifically address those operations. In considering any such findings, the Joint Commission may obtain other expert consultation.

If surveyors identify any condition that poses a threat to public or patient safety, the surveyors notify the organization's chief executive officer and Joint Commission corporate office staff. The president of the Joint Commission or, in his/her absence, a vice-president of the Joint Commission delegated by the president to do so, is authorized, on the basis of such notification or otherwise, to decide to deny accreditation and to promptly notify the organization's chief executive officer, as well as governmental authorities having jurisdiction, about this decision. The Accreditation Committee of the Board of Commissioners promptly reviews this decision to confirm or reverse it.

PUBLIC INFORMATION INTERVIEWS

Anyone who has information about an organization's compliance with the accreditation standards may request a public information interview. The Joint Commission asks the organization to provide an opportunity during a full on-site survey for the presentation of information by consumers and the public, as well as by personnel and staff of the organization undergoing survey.

The Joint Commission requires an organization to post, in a public place on its premises, the official Joint Commission announcement of the date of the survey and of the opportunity for a public information interview. Ordinarily, the public notice must be posted four weeks before the survey date; the notice must indicate that requests for a public information interview be made in writing and that the Joint Commission must receive them at least two working days before an organization's accreditation survey begins. The notice must remain posted until the first day of the survey. Furthermore, if anyone asks about the survey, the Joint Commission expects the organization to inform the person of the survey dates and of the fact that a public information interview may be requested or that such an interview is already scheduled.

The organization should promptly send any request it receives for a public information interview to the Joint Commission's Ambulatory Care Accreditation Services and retain a copy for its files. The Joint Commission acknowledges each request and sends a copy of this acknowledgment to the organization. The organization is responsible for notifying the interviewee(s) of the exact date, time, and place of the public information interview.

Surveyors are required to report on whether Joint Commission policies concerning the public information interview have been carried out properly. This includes reporting the manner in which the organization posted the notice.

Public information interviews usually are conducted during the morning of the first survey day. The organization is expected to provide reasonable accommodation either within the facility or at a conveniently accessible location near the organization. Surveyors conduct the interview session and receive the information. A representative(s) of the organization is expected to attend.

The interview consists only of the orderly receipt of information offered, verbally or in writing, within the prescribed time limit. The information is considered during the survey process and is reported to Joint Commission corporate office staff with the results and recommendations of the survey. Any further participation in the survey by an outside source of information must be authorized by the organization.

CHIEF EXECUTIVE OFFICER EXIT CONFERENCE

Joint Commission surveyors hold an exit conference with the organization's chief executive officer at the completion of all surveys. The following individuals or their designees should also attend this conference: the chairperson of the governing body, the director of nursing, the medical director, and, if applicable, the chief operating officer. The Joint Commission advises that the organization keep attendance to approximately eight people.

During the conference, the surveyors present their findings regarding any significant standards compliance problems. They also indicate, to the extent possible, the potential impact these problems will *likely* have on the final accreditation decision. The final decision regarding accreditation involves the processing of surveyor findings in accordance with specific aggregation and decision rules promulgated by the Accreditation Committee of the Joint Commission. Because of the complexity of aggregation rules, surveyors are not expected to maintain a mastery of all such rules. In addition to presenting findings and recommendations for improvement, the surveyors discuss the underlying causes of the identified problems. Organization representatives will be given an opportunity to respond to the surveyor's recommendations and to clarify issues raised by the surveyors' findings. Upon request, surveyors will also provide consultation on survey findings that may not be directly related to standards.

SUMMATION CONFERENCE

At the organization's request, the surveyors will also conduct a summation conference for all organization staff. Summation conferences are an option at initial and triennial surveys only. The purpose of this conference is to make general observations about the survey findings and, based on these findings, to indicate the organization's strengths and weaknesses. The surveyors will be available to clarify the intent of the standards and the survey process. To the extent that time permits, the surveyors will comment on acceptable methods of meeting Joint Commission standards.

ACCREDITATION DECISION AND APPEAL

Accreditation decisions are made in accordance with the accreditation and appeal procedures set out in Appendix B of this *Manual*, and these procedures are only briefly summarized here. Joint Commission staff evaluates the results of the survey, the recommendations of the surveyor(s), and any other relevant information, such as documentation of compliance with the standards, documentation of plans to correct deficiencies, or evidence of recent improvements. Using scoring guidelines and decision rules approved by the Accreditation Committee of the Board of Commissioners, staff makes a determination regarding accreditation. This determination can be for accreditation with commendation, accreditation with or without recommendations, conditional accreditation, or denial of accreditation. Recommendations are of two types. A type I recommendation is a recommendation or group of recommendations that affects the accreditation decision and should receive the highest priority in the organization's plans for improvement. Type II recommendations are supplementary or consultative in nature and do not affect the accreditation decision. They may, however, affect that decision if not dealt with appropriately by the next triennial survey. The organization's progress in resolving type I recommendations will be monitored by the Joint Commission through focused surveys, written progress reports, or both, at stated times during the accreditation cycle. Various categories of staff determinations must be reviewed by the Accreditation Committee, including, among others, all determinations to deny accreditation or to conditionally accredit if challenged by the organization.

If the Accreditation Committee determines that an organization that has not been an accredited organization during the two years prior to the survey is not entitled to an award of accreditation as a result of the survey, the organization may elect to consider the survey a consultation and education visit that does not result in an accreditation decision. If the organization makes this election, its status will be not accredited. It will be eligible for resurvey without any waiting period. An organization can only select a consultation and education option once. As stated in the following paragraph, this option does not apply in those instances where the Accreditation Committee confirms a decision of the president of the Joint Commission, or a designee, to deny accreditation to the organization because of an immediate threat to public or patient safety.

The above procedures do not apply when a surveyor identifies any condition that poses a threat to public or patient safety or other information indicates the existence of such a threat. In such cases, the president of the Joint Commission, or, in his/her absence, a vice-president of the Joint Commission delegated by the president to do so, may decide to deny accreditation to the organization. This action by the president, or his/her designee, is reported by telephone and in writing to the organization's chief executive officer and in writing to the relevant governmental authorities. The Accreditation Committee promptly reviews this decision to confirm or reverse it.

The organization has the right to pursue and have decided an appeal of any decision of the Accreditation Committee to deny accreditation before the decision becomes the final decision of the Joint Commission.

DURATION OF THE ACCREDITATION AWARD

If it is found to be in substantial compliance with Joint Commission standards, an organization is awarded accreditation for three years. The final decision to accredit an organization becomes effective as of the first day after completion of the organization's survey.

At the request of an accredited organization, the Joint Commission will conduct a full accreditation survey more frequently than once every three years. Such requests should be sent to the director of Ambulatory Care Accreditation Services.

In the process of deciding to accredit an organization, the Joint Commission determines whether survey findings warrant accreditation with any type I recommendations. When an organization is accredited subject to one or more type I recommendations, the Joint Commission monitors the organization's efforts to improve the area(s) of concern identified during the accreditation survey. An organization that receives a type I recommendation is ordinarily expected to achieve substantial or significant compliance with the relevant standard(s) within a specified time, and failure to do so can generate a decision to conditionally accredit or deny accreditation.

Monitoring by the Joint Commission and the time allotted for demonstrating improvement of an area assigned a type I recommendation depend on the nature of the concern—particularly its effect on patient care—and on the time required to satisfactorily address the concern. Organizations that receive accreditation with type I recommendations are ordinarily required to submit a written progress report or to have their compliance reviewed during an on-site survey that focuses on only those standards identified in the report as type I recommendations. Some type I recommendations, however, may require surveyors to address issues related to other standards in order to fully address compliance with the standards related to the type I recommendations. The size of the survey team and the duration of the focused survey depend on the number and extent of concerns addressed in the type I recommendations.

An accredited organization is expected to be in continuous compliance with all applicable standards and may be surveyed at any time, with or without notice to the organization, at the discretion of the Joint Commission. Such surveys are ordinarily performed in response to complaints, media coverage, or other information which may raise questions regarding compliance with standards or the adequacy of protections for patient health and safety. Failure to permit such a survey to take place can be viewed by the Joint Commission as constituting an immediate withdrawal from the accreditation program. Ordinarily, no fee is charged for a survey initiated at the Joint Commission's discretion.

The standards applied during any survey are those in effect at the time of the survey.

CONTINUING ACCREDITATION

Accreditation is not automatically renewed. An organization must undergo a full accreditation survey at least every three years, and survey findings must warrant continued accreditation. Approximately seven months before an organization's accreditation is due to expire, the Joint Commission sends the organization an Application for Survey. Following receipt of the completed application, a survey is scheduled. The Joint Commission ordinarily schedules the survey as near as possible to the organization's survey anniversary date. However, to allow latitude, surveys are ordinarily scheduled within a period beginning the month before and 60 days after the organization's anniversary date. With an organization's consent, the Joint Commission may schedule the survey more than 45 days before accreditation is due to expire.

Following a survey, an organization's previous accreditation status remains in effect until either a final decision is made to accredit or not accredit the organization.

Once an accredited organization has been surveyed, the accreditation decision-making process continues until a final accreditation decision has been reached. An organization's decision to withdraw from the accreditation process after undergoing survey and before a final accreditation decision has been made will not terminate the decision-making process; a final accreditation decision will be reached.

Accreditation is not automatically transferable, and it is not ongoing if significant changes occur in the circumstances existing at the time of the survey upon which the accreditation decision was based. If an accredited organization changes ownership or control or undergoes a significant change in its capacity or in the categories of services offered, it must notify the Joint Commission not more than 30 days after such change. Accreditation is continued until the Joint Commission can determine whether a resurvey is necessary to continue accreditation. Failure to notify the Joint Commission of ownership and services changes may result in loss of accreditation.

An accredited organization also must notify the Joint Commission not more than 30 calendar days after a merger or consolidation with another organization or before a major change in facilities or corporate structure. Under such circumstances, the Joint Commission may decide that the organization must be resurveyed. Failure to notify the Joint Commission of such changes may also result in loss of accreditation.

PUBLIC RECOGNITION

The Joint Commission provides each accredited organization with a certificate of accreditation. An organization is not charged for the initial certificate. Additional certificates can be purchased from the Joint Commission. Such requests should be sent to the Certificate Coordinator, Scheduling Department.

The certificate and all copies remain the property of the Joint Commission and must be returned to the Joint Commission if the organization is issued a new certificate reflecting a change in name, or if its accreditation expires or is withdrawn or denied for any reason.

Organizations accredited by the Joint Commission must be accurate in describing to the public the nature of their accreditation. Organizations cannot engage in any false or misleading advertising with regard to their accreditation. Any such advertising may be grounds for denial of accreditation. For example, accredited organizations cannot represent their accreditation as being awarded by the Joint Commission's corporate members (the American College of Physicians, the American College of Surgeons, the American Dental Association, the American Hospital Association, and the American Medical Association). The Joint Commission has permission to reprint the seals of its corporate members on the certificates of accreditation, but these seals must not be reproduced or displayed separately from the certificate.

QUALITY ASSESSMENT AND IMPROVEMENT

PREAMBLE

The monitoring and evaluation segment of this chapter describes the activities of a health care organization that are designed to assess and improve the quality of patient care. The section includes revisions to the 1990 standards which are intended to assist health care organizations in performing these activities more effectively. The revisions shift the emphases and further clarify certain steps in the monitoring and evaluation process.

The revised standards are based on the following principles:

- A health care organization can improve patient care and service quality—that is, increase the probability of desired patient outcomes, including patient satisfaction—by assessing and improving those governance, managerial, clinical, and support processes that most affect patient outcomes.

- Some of these processes are carried out by clinicians, some by governing body members, some by managers, and some by support personnel; some are carried out jointly by two or more of these groups.

- Whether carried out by one or more groups, the processes must be coordinated and integrated; this coordination and integration requires the attention of the managerial and clinical leaders of the organization.

- Most governance, managerial, clinical, and support staff are both motivated and competent to carry out the processes well. Therefore, the opportunities to improve the processes—and thus improve patient outcomes—are much more frequent than are mistakes and errors. Consequently, without shirking its responsibility to address serious problems involving deficits in knowledge or skill, the organization's principal goal should be to help everyone improve the processes in which he/she is involved.

These principles underlie the continuous assessment and improvement of quality. For ambulatory care organizations, the natural next step in the steady progression of approaches from implicit peer review to audits to systematic quality assurance (QA) is to continuous improvement.

Beginning with this 1992 *Manual* and progressing over the next few years, the Joint Commission is incrementally revising the standards on quality assessment and improvement to help health care organizations use their current commitment, resources, and approaches to improving patient care quality more effectively and efficiently. The revisions in this *Manual* are designed to encourage organizations to evaluate their current activities in light of the above principles, and to assist those organizations that are already moving toward an approach to continuously improve quality. In subsequent editions of this *Manual*, the standards revisions will begin to establish expectations for all health care organizations to continuously improve quality.

The revisions in the monitoring and evaluation standards are intended to shift some emphases to help health care organizations overcome common weaknesses in current QA practice which can inhibit the development of an approach to continuously improving quality. These common weaknesses in current practice include

- frequently focusing on only the clinical aspects of care, rather than on the full series of interrelated governance, managerial, support, and clinical processes that affect patient outcomes;

- frequently compartmentalizing QA activities in accordance with organizational structure (for example, by program, by discipline), rather than organizing quality improvement activities around the flow of patient care, in which the interrelated processes are often cross-disciplinary and cross-program;

- frequently focusing only on the performance of individuals, especially on problem performance, rather than on how well the processes in which they participate are performed, how well the processes are coordinated and integrated (for example, the "handoffs"), and how the processes can be improved;

- frequently initiating action only when a problem is identified, rather than also trying to find better ways to carry out processes; and

- separating the appropriateness ("Was the right thing done?") and effectiveness ("Was it done right?") of care from the efficiency of care, rather than integrating efforts to improve patient outcomes with those to improve efficiency (that is, improving value).

Because of its frequent, exclusive focus on individual performance, especially problem performance, current QA practice often has a negative connotation. This can interfere with health care professionals' instinct to pursue lifelong self-assessment and continuous personal growth.

The changes in the monitoring and evaluation standards are designed to shift the emphases of quality assessment and improvement activities away from an approach that is frequently (1) program and discipline specific, (2) exclusively direct care focused, and (3) individual and problem oriented to an approach that reflects the principles described above. This approach is expected to better promote the professional instinct for continuous improvement.

Please note that the phrase "monitoring and evaluation of the quality and appropriateness of care" has been modified in Required Characteristics QA.1.6.1 through AZ.1.6.2.10.3 by deleting "and appropriateness," since contemporary definitions of quality include appropriateness among its characteristics (for example, effectiveness, appropriateness, accessibility, continuity, efficiency).

STANDARD

QA.1   There is an ongoing quality assessment and improvement program designed to objectively and systematically monitor and evaluate the quality and appropriateness of patient care, pursue opportunities to improve patient care, and resolve identified problems.*   1 2 3 4 5 NA

REQUIRED CHARACTERISTICS

QA.1.1   The governing body strives to assure high-quality patient care by requiring and supporting the establishment and maintenance of an effective organizationwide quality assessment and improvement program.*   1 2 3 4 5 NA

Note: For an explanation of the rating scale, see "Using the Manual," page ix.

*All asterisked items are key factors in the accreditation decision process. For an explanation of the use of key factors, see "Using the Manual," page ix.

QA.1.2 Clinical and administrative staffs monitor and evaluate the quality and appropriateness of patient care and clinical performance, resolve identified problems, and report information to the governing body that the governing body needs to assist it in fulfilling its responsibility for the quality of patient care.*   1 2 3 4 5 NA

QA.1.3 There is a written plan for the quality assessment and improvement program that describes the program's objectives, organization, scope, and mechanisms for overseeing the effectiveness of monitoring, evaluation, and problem-solving activities.*   1 2 3 4 5 NA

QA.1.4 The implementation of the quality assessment and improvement program is the responsibility of a designated individual or group.*   1 2 3 4 5 NA

QA.1.5 The scope of the quality assessment and improvement program includes at least the activities listed in Required Characteristics QA.1.5.1 through QA.1.5.9 and described in or related to other chapters of this *Manual.*   1 2 3 4 5 NA

QA.1.5.1 The quality and appropriateness of diagnostic and treatment procedures are evaluated (see "Quality of Care" Required Characteristics QC.1.1.5 and QC.1.1.6)*;   1 2 3 4 5 NA

QA.1.5.2 The quality, content, and completeness of medical record entries are evaluated (see "Quality of Care" Required Characteristic QC.1.1.8)*;   1 2 3 4 5 NA

QA.1.5.3 Clinical performance is evaluated (see "Quality of Care" chapter)*;   1 2 3 4 5 NA

QA.1.5.4 The use of medications is reviewed (see "Pharmaceutical Services" Required Characteristic PS.1.6)*;   1 2 3 4 5 NA

QA.1.5.5 Patient satisfaction is evaluated (see "Administration" Required Characteristic AD.1.3)*;   1 2 3 4 5 NA

QA.1.5.6 The quality and appropriateness of surgical and anesthesia services, when provided, are evaluated (see "Surgical and Anesthesia Services" Required Characteristic SA.1.20)*;   1 2 3 4 5 NA

QA.1.5.7 The cases of patients who require hospitalization following ambulatory surgery are reviewed (see "Surgical and Anesthesia Services" Required Characteristic SA.1.20.1)*;   1 2 3 4 5 NA

QA.1.5.8 The quality and appropriateness of emergency services, when provided, are evaluated (see "Emergency Services" Required Characteristic ES.1.12)*; and   1 2 3 4 5 NA

QA.1.5.9 There is quality control in pathology and laboratory services, and in radiology services, when provided (see "Laboratory Services and Pathology" Required Characteristic LP.1.2.4 and "Radiology Services" Required Characteristic RS.1.8).*   1 2 3 4 5 NA

QA.1.6 Monitoring and evaluation activities, including those described in Required Characteristics QA.1.5.1 through QA.1.5.9 reflect the activities described in Required Characteristics QA.1.6.1 through QA.1.6.2.10.3.   1 2 3 4 5 NA

All asterisked items are key factors in the accreditation decision process. For an explanation of the use of key factors, see "Using the Manual," page ix.

QA.1.6.1   There is a planned, systematic, and ongoing process for monitoring, evaluating, and improving the quality of care and of key governance, managerial, and support activities which has the characteristics described in Required Characteristics QA.1.6.2 through QA.1.6.2.10.3.*   1 2 3 4 5 NA

QA.1.6.2   Those aspects of care that are most important to the health and safety of the patients served are identified.*   1 2 3 4 5 NA

QA.1.6.2.1   These important aspects of care are those that

QA.1.6.2.1.1   occur frequently or affect large numbers of patients*;   1 2 3 4 5 NA

QA.1.6.2.1.2   place patients at risk of serious consequences or of deprivation of substantial benefit when*   1 2 3 4 5 NA

QA.1.6.2.1.2.1   the care is not provided correctly,* or   1 2 3 4 5 NA

QA.1.6.2.1.2.2   the care is not provided when indicated,* or   1 2 3 4 5 NA

QA.1.6.2.1.2.3   the care is provided when not indicated*; and/or   1 2 3 4 5 NA

QA.1.6.2.1.3   tend to produce problems for patients or staff.*   1 2 3 4 5 NA

QA.1.6.2.2   Indicators are identified to monitor the quality of important aspects of care.*   1 2 3 4 5 NA

QA.1.6.2.2.1   The indicators are related to the quality of care and may include clinical criteria (sometimes called "clinical standards," "practice guidelines," or "practice parameters").*   1 2 3 4 5 NA

QA.1.6.2.2.1.1   The indicators are

QA.1.6.2.2.1.1.1   objective,*   1 2 3 4 5 NA

QA.1.6.2.2.1.1.2   measurable,* and   1 2 3 4 5 NA

QA.1.6.2.2.1.1.3   based on current knowledge and clinical experience.*   1 2 3 4 5 NA

QA.1.6.2.3   Data are collected for each indicator.*   1 2 3 4 5 NA

QA.1.6.2.3.1   The frequency of data collection for each indicator and the sampling of events or activities is related to

QA.1.6.2.3.1.1   the frequency of the event or activity monitored*;   1 2 3 4 5 NA

QA.1.6.2.3.1.2   the significance of the event or activity monitored*; and   1 2 3 4 5 NA

QA.1.6.2.3.1.3   the extent to which the important aspect of care monitored by the indicator has been demonstrated to be problem free.*   1 2 3 4 5 NA

QA.1.6.2.4   The data collected for each indicator are organized so that situations in which an evaluation of the quality of care is indicated are readily identified.*   1 2 3 4 5 NA

QA.1.6.2.4.1   Such evaluations are prompted by

QA.1.6.2.4.1.1   important single clinical events* and   1 2 3 4 5 NA

---

*All asterisked items are key factors in the accreditation decision process. For an explanation of the use of key factors, see "Using the Manual," page ix.

QA.1.6.2.4.1.2   levels or patterns/trends in care or outcomes that are at significant variance with predetermined levels and/or patterns/trends in care or outcomes.*   1 2 3 4 5 NA

QA.1.6.2.4.2   Such evaluations may also be initiated by comparison of the organization's performance with that of other organizations ("benchmarking").*   1 2 3 4 5 NA

QA.1.6.2.4.3   Such evaluations may also be initiated when there is a desire to improve overall performance.*   1 2 3 4 5 NA

QA.1.6.2.5   When initiated, the evaluation of an important aspect of care

QA.1.6.2.5.1   includes a more detailed analysis of patterns/trends in the data collected on the indicators*;   1 2 3 4 5 NA

QA.1.6.2.5.2   is designed to identify opportunities to improve, or problems in, the quality of care*; and   1 2 3 4 5 NA

QA.1.6.2.5.3   includes review by peers when analysis of the care provided by a practitioner is undertaken.*   1 2 3 4 5 NA

QA.1.6.2.6   When an important opportunity to improve, or a problem in, the quality of care is identified,

QA.1.6.2.6.1   action is taken to improve the care or correct the problem* and   1 2 3 4 5 NA

QA.1.6.2.6.2   the effectiveness of the action taken is assessed through continued monitoring of the care.*   1 2 3 4 5 NA

QA.1.6.2.7   The findings, conclusions, recommendations, actions taken, and results of the actions taken are

QA.1.6.2.7.1   documented* and   1 2 3 4 5 NA

QA.1.6.2.7.2   reported through established channels.*   1 2 3 4 5 NA

QA.1.6.2.8   Relevant results from the monitoring and evaluation activity

QA.1.6.2.8.1   are used primarily to study and improve processes that affect patient care outcomes* and,   1 2 3 4 5 NA

QA.1.6.2.8.2   when relevant to the performance of an individual, are used as a component of the evaluation of individual capabilities.*   1 2 3 4 5 NA

QA.1.6.2.9   As part of the annual reappraisal of the organization's quality assessment and improvement program, the effectiveness of the monitoring and evaluation process is assessed.*   1 2 3 4 5 NA

QA.1.6.2.10   Each department/service/program participates in

QA.1.6.2.10.1   the identification of the important aspects of care or services for the department/service/program*;   1 2 3 4 5 NA

QA.1.6.2.10.2   the identification of the indicators used to monitor the quality of the important aspects of care*; and   1 2 3 4 5 NA

QA.1.6.2.10.3   the evaluation of the quality of care.*   1 2 3 4 5 NA

All asterisked items are key factors in the accreditation decision process. For an explanation of the use of key factors, see "Using the Manual," page ix.

QA.1.7   The administration and coordination of the organization's overall quality assessment and improvement program are designed to assure that
the activities described in Required Characteristics QA.1.7.1 through
QA.1.7.5 are undertaken.   1 2 3 4 5 NA

QA.1.7.1   Each of the monitoring and evaluation activities outlined in
Required Characteristics QA.1.5.1 through QA.1.6.2.10.3 is performed
appropriately and effectively.   1 2 3 4 5 NA

QA.1.7.2   Necessary information is communicated among departments,
services, or programs when opportunities to improve, or problems in,
patient care involve more than one department, service, or program.*   1 2 3 4 5 NA

QA.1.7.3   The status of identified problems is tracked to assure improvement or resolution.*   1 2 3 4 5 NA

QA.1.7.4   Information from departments, services, or programs and
the findings of discrete quality assessment and improvement activities
are used to detect trends, patterns of performance, or potential problems
that affect more than one department, service, or program.*   1 2 3 4 5 NA

QA.1.7.5   The objectives, scope, organization, and effectiveness of the
quality assessment and improvement program are evaluated at least
annually and revised as necessary.*   1 2 3 4 5 NA

COMMENTS AND RECOMMENDATIONS

Use this space to explain each 2, 3, 4, or 5 rating and to specify methods for better
meeting the intent of the standard.

*All asterisked items are key factors in the accreditation decision process. For an explanation of the
use of key factors, see "Using the Manual," page ix.*

QUALITY OF CARE

STANDARD

QC.1 The organization delivers health services that demonstrate a high quality of care. These services are provided in a manner consistent with principles of professional practice and reflect concern for the acceptability, accessibility, availability, and cost of services.   1 2 3 4 5 NA

REQUIRED CHARACTERISTICS

QC.1.1 The provision of high-quality health care services is demonstrated by at least the following: 1 2 3 4 5 NA

QC.1.1.1 Available and accessible health services*;   1 2 3 4 5 NA

QC.1.1.2 A description of the intake system for patients during and after normal hours of operation;   1 2 3 4 5 NA

QC.1.1.3 Provision for, and information about, emergency and after-hours care*;   1 2 3 4 5 NA

QC.1.1.4 A mechanism for informing patients of the names, professions, and titles of the professionals providing and/or responsible for their care*;   1 2 3 4 5 NA

QC.1.1.5 The use of appropriate diagnostic procedures, including laboratory and radiology studies when indicated*;   1 2 3 4 5 NA

QC.1.1.6 Treatment that is consistent with the clinical impression or working diagnosis*;   1 2 3 4 5 NA

QC.1.1.7 The availability and use of appropriate consultation*;   1 2 3 4 5 NA

QC.1.1.8 Appropriate, accurate, and complete medical record entries;   1 2 3 4 5 NA

QC.1.1.9 Patient instruction and education regarding the treatment program, including the use of medications and therapies*;   1 2 3 4 5 NA

QC.1.1.10 Timely and adequate transfer of appropriate patient care documents and information when patients are transferred to or from other health care providers within and/or outside the organization*;   1 2 3 4 5 NA

QC.1.1.10.1 The transfer of information includes any advance directives given by the patient to the ambulatory care organization.*   1 2 3 4 5 NA

QC.1.1.11 Documents and other evidence of continuity of care*;   1 2 3 4 5 NA

QC.1.1.12 Reasonable follow-up regarding patient adherence to a plan of care*;   1 2 3 4 5 NA

Note: *For an explanation of the rating scale, see "Using the Manual," page ix.*

All asterisked items are key factors in the accreditation decision process. For an explanation of the use of key factors, see "Using the Manual," page ix.

QC.1.1.13   A system for timely identification and notification of those patients who require additional follow-up for significant problems or illnesses, including results of laboratory and radiology studies*;   1 2 3 4 5 NA

QC.1.1.14   Procedures, including adequate surveillance techniques, that minimize sources of and transmission of infections*;   1 2 3 4 5 NA

QC.1.1.15   The availability of resources to respond to medical emergencies that may arise in connection with the services provided to patients*; and   1 2 3 4 5 NA

QC.1.1.16   Emergency carts that are kept in adequate and proper supply.*   1 2 3 4 5 NA

   QC.1.1.16.1   Written policies address the timely review and inspection of each cart.   1 2 3 4 5 NA

QC.1.2   Concern for the cost of care is demonstrated by the

QC.1.2.1   relevance of health care services to the needs of patients*;   1 2 3 4 5 NA

QC.1.2.2   absence of duplicative diagnostic procedures;   1 2 3 4 5 NA

QC.1.2.3   appropriateness of treatment frequency;   1 2 3 4 5 NA

QC.1.2.4   use of the least expensive alternative resources when suitable;   1 2 3 4 5 NA

QC.1.2.5   use of ancillary services consistent with patients' needs; and   1 2 3 4 5 NA

QC.1.2.6   evaluation of cost-benefit factors by appropriate medical personnel to determine which, if any, routine laboratory and x-ray studies are required.   1 2 3 4 5 NA

COMMENTS AND RECOMMENDATIONS

Use this space to explain each 2, 3, 4, or 5 rating and to specify methods for better meeting the intent of the standard.

All asterisked items are key factors in the accreditation decision process. For an explanation of the use of key factors, see "Using the Manual," page ix.

MEDICAL RECORDS

STANDARD

MR.1 The organization maintains a medical record system that permits prompt retrieval of information. Medical records are legible, documented accurately in a timely manner, and readily accessible to health care practitioners.*

1 2 3 4 5 NA

REQUIRED CHARACTERISTICS

MR.1.1 The organization develops and maintains a system for the collection, processing, maintenance, storage, retrieval, and distribution of medical records.*

1 2 3 4 5 NA

MR.1.2 All clinical information relevant to a patient is readily available to the health care practitioner staff.*

1 2 3 4 5 NA

MR.1.2.1 This information includes any advance directives given by the patient to the ambulatory care organization.*

1 2 3 4 5 NA

MR.1.3 Except as required by law, any record that contains clinical, social, financial, or other data on a particular patient is treated in a strictly confidential manner and is reasonably protected from loss, tampering, alteration, destruction, and unauthorized or inadvertent disclosure of information.*

1 2 3 4 5 NA

MR.1.4 An individual is in charge of medical records.*

1 2 3 4 5 NA

MR.1.4.1 This individual's responsibilities include, but need not be limited to,

MR.1.4.1.1 maintaining the confidentiality, security, and physical safety of the patients' medical records*;

1 2 3 4 5 NA

MR.1.4.1.2 maintaining the unique identification of each patient's medical record;

1 2 3 4 5 NA

MR.1.4.1.3 supervising the collection, processing, maintenance, storage, timely retrieval, and distribution of medical records; and

1 2 3 4 5 NA

MR.1.4.1.4 maintaining a predetermined, organized medical record format.*

1 2 3 4 5 NA

MR.1.5 Written policies concerning medical records address, but need not be limited to, the following:

MR.1.5.1 The confidentiality of patient information contained in each medical record*;

1 2 3 4 5 NA

Note: For an explanation of the rating scale, see "Using the Manual," page ix.

*All asterisked items are key factors in the accreditation decision process. For an explanation of the use of key factors, see "Using the Manual," page ix.

MR.1.5.2   The mechanisms used to safeguard each medical record from loss, tampering, alteration, or destruction*;   1 2 3 4 5 NA

MR.1.5.3   The retention of active medical records*;   1 2 3 4 5 NA

MR.1.5.4   The retirement of inactive medical records*;   1 2 3 4 5 NA

MR.1.5.5   The timely entry of data into the medical records*;   1 2 3 4 5 NA

MR.1.5.6   The release of information contained in medical records*; and   1 2 3 4 5 NA

MR.1.5.7   Any requirement concerning consent for treatment.*   1 2 3 4 5 NA

MR.1.6   Except as required by law, the content and format of medical records are maintained in a uniform manner.*   1 2 3 4 5 NA

MR.1.7   Reports of histories and physical examinations, progress notes, and other materials—such as laboratory reports, x-ray readings, and consultations—are incorporated into each patient's medical record in a timely manner.*   1 2 3 4 5 NA

MR.1.8   Medical records are available to health care practitioner staff any time the organization is open to patients.*   1 2 3 4 5 NA

MR.1.9   To facilitate the ongoing provision of care, there is a list of known significant diagnoses, conditions, procedures, drug allergies, and medications in the record of each patient who receives continuing ambulatory services.*   1 2 3 4 5 NA

MR.1.9.1   The list includes at least the following items:

MR.1.9.1.1   known significant medical diagnoses and conditions*;   1 2 3 4 5 NA

MR.1.9.1.2   known significant surgical and invasive procedures*;   1 2 3 4 5 NA

MR.1.9.1.3   known adverse and allergic reactions to drugs*; and   1 2 3 4 5 NA

MR.1.9.1.4   medications known to be prescribed for and/or used by the patient.*   1 2 3 4 5 NA

MR.1.9.2   The list is initiated and maintained for each patient by the third visit.*   1 2 3 4 5 NA

MR.1.9.2.1   The initial list includes items based on any initial medical history and physical examination.*   1 2 3 4 5 NA

MR.1.9.2.2   The list is updated on subsequent visits with additional information pertaining to the items specified in Required Characteristics MR.1.9.1.1 to MR.1.9.1.4.*   1 2 3 4 5 NA

MR.1.9.2.2.1   Each item is dated to facilitate locating relevant information in the medical record.*   1 2 3 4 5 NA

MR.1.9.2.2.2   When significant information concerning the patient is located in another record, a written notation at the relevant item in the list indicates where the other information is located.*   1 2 3 4 5 NA

MR.1.9.2.2.3   Updates need not repeat diagnoses or conditions that recur during ongoing treatment.

MR.1.9.3   The list is located in the same place in every patient's medical record.*   1 2 3 4 5 NA

All asterisked items are key factors in the accreditation decision process. For an explanation of the use of key factors, see "Using the Manual," page ix.

MR.1.9.3.1 Each practitioner in the organization is informed of the location of the list.	1 2 3 4 5 NA

MR.1.10   For each visit, at least the following information is entered in the patient's medical record*:

MR.1.10.1 Date;	1 2 3 4 5 NA
MR.1.10.2 Department (if the organization is departmentalized);	1 2 3 4 5 NA
MR.1.10.3 Practitioner's name and profession (for example, PT, MD, RN, DDS, DMD);	1 2 3 4 5 NA
MR.1.10.4 Chief complaint or purpose of visit*;	1 2 3 4 5 NA
MR.1.10.5 Objective findings*;	1 2 3 4 5 NA
MR.1.10.6 Diagnosis or medical impression*;	1 2 3 4 5 NA
MR.1.10.7 Studies ordered, such as laboratory or x-ray studies*;	1 2 3 4 5 NA
MR.1.10.8 Therapies administered*;	1 2 3 4 5 NA
MR.1.10.9 Disposition, recommendations, and instructions to patients*; and	1 2 3 4 5 NA
MR.1.10.10 Signatures or initials of practitioners.*	1 2 3 4 5 NA

MR.1.11 Medical record entries are legible to clinical personnel.	1 2 3 4 5 NA
MR.1.12 Any notation in a patient's medical record indicating diagnostic or therapeutic intervention as part of clinical research is clearly contrasted with entries that are made with regard to the provision of care.	1 2 3 4 5 NA
MR.1.13 When a patient was treated elsewhere—such as at a hospital, ambulatory surgical facility, nursing home, or physician's or consultant's office—clinical summaries or other pertinent documents are obtained when necessary for promoting continuity of care.*	1 2 3 4 5 NA

COMMENTS AND RECOMMENDATIONS

Use this space to explain each 2, 3, 4, or 5 rating and to specify methods for better meeting the intent of the standard.

All asterisked items are key factors in the accreditation decision process. For an explanation of the use of key factors, see "Using the Manual," page ix.

RIGHTS AND RESPONSIBILITIES OF PATIENTS

STANDARD

RP.1   Patients are treated in a manner that recognizes their basic human rights.*   1 2 3 4 5 NA

REQUIRED CHARACTERISTICS

RP.1.1   The organization has a written policy on the rights and responsibilities of patients.*   1 2 3 4 5 NA

RP.1.1.1   This policy includes those rights specified in Required Characteristics RP.1.2 through RP.1.5.2.1.   1 2 3 4 5 NA

RP.1.2   Patients are treated with respect, consideration, and dignity.*   1 2 3 4 5 NA

RP.1.3   Patients are assured confidential treatment of disclosures and records and are afforded the opportunity to approve or refuse the release of such information, except when release is required by law.*   1 2 3 4 5 NA

RP.1.4   Patients are provided, to the degree known, information concerning their diagnoses, treatments, and prognoses.*   1 2 3 4 5 NA

RP.1.4.1   When concern for a patient's health makes it inadvisable to give such information to the patient, such information is made available to an individual designated by the patient or to a legally authorized individual.*   1 2 3 4 5 NA

RP.1.5   Patients are given the opportunity to participate in decisions involving their health care, unless this is contraindicated by concerns for the patient's health.*   1 2 3 4 5 NA

RP.1.5.1   In an organization that provides primary/continuing care, mechanisms are in place to assist in the development of advance directives for future care for those patients who request such assistance.   1 2 3 4 5 NA

RP.1.5.1.1   In an organization that does not provide primary/continuing care, policies and procedures address the organization's response to advance directives.   1 2 3 4 5 NA

RP.1.5.2   The organization's policies and procedures support the right of the patient to participate in decisions about the intensity and scope of treatment to be provided within the limits of the organization's philosophy and mission and applicable law and regulation.   1 2 3 4 5 NA

Note: *For an explanation of the rating scale, see "Using the Manual," page ix.*

All asterisked items are key factors in the accreditation decision process. For an explanation of the use of key factors, see "Using the Manual," page ix.

RP.1.5.2.1 Policies and procedures regarding the care of the terminally ill patient support the participation of the patient in decisions regarding pain and symptom management and acknowledge the psychosocial and spiritual needs of the patient and the family regarding the patient's terminal illness.   1 2 3 4 5 NA

RP.1.6 The policy regarding patients' rights and responsibilities includes provisions designed to resolve complaints relating to the quality of care.*   1 2 3 4 5 NA

RP.1.6.1 The organization has a mechanism for receiving and responding to patients' and families' complaints concerning the quality of care.*   1 2 3 4 5 NA

RP.1.6.1.1 Patients and families are informed of their right to present complaints and of how to do so.*   1 2 3 4 5 NA

RP.1.6.1.2 The organization analyzes the complaint, and, when indicated, takes appropriate corrective action.*   1 2 3 4 5 NA

RP.1.6.1.3 Each patient or family making a significant complaint receives a response from the organization which substantively addresses the complaint.*   1 2 3 4 5 NA

RP.1.6.1.4 Presentation of a complaint does not in itself serve to compromise a patient's future access to care.*   1 2 3 4 5 NA

RP.1.7 Information is available to patients and staff concerning the

RP.1.7.1 policy on the rights and responsibilities of patients*;   1 2 3 4 5 NA

RP.1.7.2 services available at the organization*;   1 2 3 4 5 NA

RP.1.7.3 provisions made for after-hours and emergency coverage*;   1 2 3 4 5 NA

RP.1.7.4 conduct and responsibilities of patients, including the consequences of refusing treatment or not complying with therapy*;   1 2 3 4 5 NA

RP.1.7.5 policy on treatment of an unemancipated minor not accompanied by an adult*;   1 2 3 4 5 NA

RP.1.7.6 right to refuse to participate in experimental research*;   1 2 3 4 5 NA

RP.1.7.7 fees for services*;   1 2 3 4 5 NA

RP.1.7.8 policies concerning payment of fees*; and   1 2 3 4 5 NA

RP.1.7.9 resources available for voicing grievances to the organization's staff and governing body and for recommending changes in policies and services.*   1 2 3 4 5 NA

RP.1.8 A procedure for reporting public health concerns to the appropriate authorities is established.*   1 2 3 4 5 NA

RP.1.9 There is a means of communicating in the languages of the population groups for which the services of the organization are intended.*   1 2 3 4 5 NA

All asterisked items are key factors in the accreditation decision process. For an explanation of the use of key factors, see "Using the Manual," page ix.

COMMENTS AND RECOMMENDATIONS

Use this space to explain each 2, 3, 4, or 5 rating and to specify methods for better meeting the intent of the standard.

GOVERNING BODY

STANDARD

GB.1   The organization has a governing body that sets policy and has overall
responsibility for the organization.*   1 2 3 4 5 NA

REQUIRED CHARACTERISTICS

GB.1.1   The organization is a legally constituted entity in the state(s) in which it
is located and in which it provides services.*   1 2 3 4 5 NA

GB.1.1.1   The organization is constituted by at least one of the following:

GB.1.1.1.1   Charter,   1 2 3 4 5 NA

GB.1.1.1.2   Articles of incorporation,   1 2 3 4 5 NA

GB.1.1.1.3   Partnership agreement,   1 2 3 4 5 NA

GB.1.1.1.4   Franchise agreement, and/or   1 2 3 4 5 NA

GB.1.1.1.5   Legislative or executive act.   1 2 3 4 5 NA

GB.1.2   The governing body makes full disclosure of ownership.*   1 2 3 4 5 NA

GB.1.2.1   The names and addresses of all owners or controlling parties—whether individuals, partnerships, trusts, corporate bodies, or
subdivisions of other bodies, such as public agencies or religious,
fraternal, or other philanthropic organizations—are made known.   1 2 3 4 5 NA

GB.1.2.2   For corporations, the names and addresses of officers, directors, and principal stockholders, either beneficial or of record, are
disclosed.   1 2 3 4 5 NA

GB.1.2.3   Accredited organizations notify the Joint Commission within
30 days following any change in ownership that involves a majority
interest.*   1 2 3 4 5 NA

GB.1.3   The governing body has the overall responsibility and authority for the
operation and performance of the organization.*   1 2 3 4 5 NA

GB.1.3.1   Responsibilities of the governing body are documented.*   1 2 3 4 5 NA

GB.1.3.1.1   These responsibilities include, but need not be limited
to, the following:

GB.1.3.1.1.1   Adopting a statement of the mission, goals, and
objectives of the organization, which includes a description of the
services provided*;   1 2 3 4 5 NA

Note: *For an explanation of the rating scale, see "Using the Manual," page ix.*

**All asterisked items are key factors in the accreditation decision process. For an explanation of the
use of key factors, see "Using the Manual," page ix.*

GB.1.3.1.1.2 Establishing an organizational structure and specifying functional relationships among the various components of the organization*;   1 2 3 4 5 NA

GB.1.3.1.1.3 Adopting bylaws or similar rules and regulations to establish authority and responsibility and to provide for the orderly development and management of the organization*;   1 2 3 4 5 NA

GB.1.3.1.1.4 Adopting such policies or procedures as may be necessary for the orderly conduct of the organization*;   1 2 3 4 5 NA

GB.1.3.1.1.5 Adopting a program to evaluate the quality of care provided and to appropriately address identified problems in care*;   1 2 3 4 5 NA

GB.1.3.1.1.6 Reviewing and taking appropriate action on all matters relating to the legal conduct of the organization and its staff*;   1 2 3 4 5 NA

GB.1.3.1.1.7 Establishing a system of financial management and accountability*;   1 2 3 4 5 NA

GB.1.3.1.1.8 Establishing a policy on the rights and responsibilities of patients*;   1 2 3 4 5 NA

GB.1.3.1.1.9 Approving, with review as appropriate by the professional staff, all major contracts or arrangements affecting the medical care provided under its auspices, including, but not necessarily limited to,*   1 2 3 4 5 NA

GB.1.3.1.1.9.1 the employment of practitioners,*   1 2 3 4 5 NA

GB.1.3.1.1.9.2 the provision of radiology services and pathology and medical laboratory services,*   1 2 3 4 5 NA

GB.1.3.1.1.9.3 the use of external laboratories,*   1 2 3 4 5 NA

GB.1.3.1.1.9.4 the provision of care by other organizations,* and   1 2 3 4 5 NA

GB.1.3.1.1.9.5 the provision of education for students and postgraduate trainees*;   1 2 3 4 5 NA

GB.1.3.1.1.10 Formulating long-range plans in accordance with the mission and goals of the organization; and   1 2 3 4 5 NA

GB.1.3.1.1.11 Operating the organization without limitation by reason of race, creed, sex, or national origin.*   1 2 3 4 5 NA

GB.1.4 The governing body meets at least annually and keeps such minutes or other records as may be necessary to demonstrate the ongoing discharge of its responsibilities.*   1 2 3 4 5 NA

GB.1.5 The governing body elects, appoints, or employs officers and/or administrators to direct the clinical and administrative activities of the organization.*   1 2 3 4 5 NA

GB.1.5.1 The authority, responsibility, and function of such positions are clearly and specifically documented.   1 2 3 4 5 NA

All asterisked items are key factors in the accreditation decision process. For an explanation of the use of key factors, see "Using the Manual," page ix.

GB.1.6   The governing body makes initial appointments and reappointments and grants or curtails delineated clinical privileges based on documented peer advice and recommendations from appropriate professional staff.*   1 2 3 4 5 NA

GB.1.6.1   Such actions are based on documented evidence of the following and are consistent with applicable law*:   1 2 3 4 5 NA

GB.1.6.1.1   Education,   1 2 3 4 5 NA

GB.1.6.1.2   Training,   1 2 3 4 5 NA

GB.1.6.1.3   Experience, and   1 2 3 4 5 NA

GB.1.6.1.4   Competence of the health care practitioner, as indicated in part by relevant findings of quality assessment and improvement activities and other reasonable indicators of current qualifications.*   1 2 3 4 5 NA

GB.1.6.2   Each practitioner providing patient care services under the auspices of the organization without supervision or direction does so in accordance with delineated clinical privileges granted by the governing body.*   1 2 3 4 5 NA

GB.1.6.2.1   The clinical privileges are specific to the practitioner and the care the practitioner provides within the organization.*   1 2 3 4 5 NA

GB.1.6.2.2   The clinical privileges are reviewed and renewed, revised, or curtailed at a minimum interval that does not exceed two years and that is specified in the governing body bylaws or policies.*   1 2 3 4 5 NA

GB.1.7   The governing body encourages personnel to participate in continuing education that is relevant to their responsibilities.   1 2 3 4 5 NA

COMMENTS AND RECOMMENDATIONS

Use this space to explain each 2, 3, 4, or 5 rating and to specify methods for better meeting the intent of the standard.

All asterisked items are key factors in the accreditation decision process. For an explanation of the use of key factors, see "Using the Manual," page ix.

ADMINISTRATION

STANDARD

AD.1   The organization is administered in a manner that promotes the provision of high-quality health services and fulfills the organization's mission, goals, and objectives.*

1 2 3 4 5 NA

REQUIRED CHARACTERISTICS

AD.1.1   Administrative policies, procedures, and controls are established, implemented, and reviewed at least annually to promote the orderly and efficient management of the organization.*

1 2 3 4 5 NA

AD.1.1.1   These policies, procedures, and controls address at least the following:

AD.1.1.1.1   Enforcing those policies delegated by the governing body *;

1 2 3 4 5 NA

AD.1.1.1.2   Employing qualified management personnel*;

1 2 3 4 5 NA

AD.1.1.1.3   Employing a sufficient number of competent, appropriately trained or educated, and supervised personnel to adequately support the organization's clinical and management objectives*;

1 2 3 4 5 NA

AD.1.1.1.4   Forecasting and planning for the needs of the organization, as determined by the governing body;

1 2 3 4 5 NA

AD.1.1.1.5   Taking all reasonable steps to comply with applicable laws and regulations*;

1 2 3 4 5 NA

AD.1.1.1.6   Protecting the organization's assets*;

1 2 3 4 5 NA

AD.1.1.1.7   Implementing fiscal controls, including, but not necessarily limited to,

1 2 3 4 5 NA

AD.1.1.1.7.1   authorization and record procedures to provide accounting controls over all assets, liabilities, revenues, and expenses,

1 2 3 4 5 NA

AD.1.1.1.7.2   policies and procedures for controlling accounts receivable and accounts payable and for handling cash and credit arrangements, and

1 2 3 4 5 NA

AD.1.1.1.7.3   rates and charges for services;

1 2 3 4 5 NA

AD.1.1.1.8   Using methods of communicating and reporting that are designed to promote the orderly flow of information within the organization;

1 2 3 4 5 NA

Note: *For an explanation of the rating scale, see "Using the Manual," page ix.*

All asterisked items are key factors in the accreditation decision process. For an explanation of the use of key factors, see "Using the Manual," page ix.

AD.1.1.1.9   Controlling the purchase, maintenance, and distribution of the organization's equipment, materials, and facilities*;   1 2 3 4 5 NA

AD.1.1.1.10   Establishing lines of authority and accountability that provide for appropriate supervision of personnel*; and   1 2 3 4 5 NA

AD.1.1.1.11   Establishing controls relating to the custody of the official documents of the organization.*   1 2 3 4 5 NA

AD.1.2   Written personnel policies and procedures are established and implemented to facilitate attainment of the organization's goals and objectives.*   1 2 3 4 5 NA

AD.1.2.1   These policies and procedures are explained and available to employees at the time of their employment.   1 2 3 4 5 NA

AD.1.2.2   Personnel policies require

AD.1.2.2.1   current, written job descriptions that delineate functional responsibilities and authority*;   1 2 3 4 5 NA

AD.1.2.2.2   the employment of personnel who have qualifications commensurate with job responsibilities and authority, including appropriate licensure or certification*; and   1 2 3 4 5 NA

AD.1.2.2.3   periodic appraisal of each individual's job performance.*   1 2 3 4 5 NA

AD.1.2.2.3.1   Relevant findings of quality assessment and improvement activities are reviewed as part of the performance appraisals of those individuals who provide direct patient services in the organization.*   1 2 3 4 5 NA

AD.1.3   The organization periodically assesses patient satisfaction with the facilities and services provided.*   1 2 3 4 5 NA

AD.1.3.1   The findings of this assessment are reviewed by the governing body.*   1 2 3 4 5 NA

AD.1.3.2   When appropriate, the findings are incorporated into the quality assessment and improvement program.*   1 2 3 4 5 NA

AD.1.4   When students and postgraduate trainees are present, their status is defined in the organization's personnel policies.*   1 2 3 4 5 NA

All asterisked items are key factors in the accreditation decision process. For an explanation of the use of key factors, see "Using the Manual," page ix.

COMMENTS AND RECOMMENDATIONS

Use this space to explain each 2, 3, 4, or 5 rating and to specify methods for better meeting the intent of the standard.

PLANT, TECHNOLOGY, AND SAFETY MANAGEMENT

STANDARD

PL.1   There is a safety management program that is designed to provide a physical environment free of hazards and to manage staff activities to reduce the risk of human injury.*   1 2 3 4 5 NA

REQUIRED CHARACTERISTICS

PL.1.1   The governing body strives to assure a safe environment for patients, personnel, and visitors by requiring and supporting the establishment and maintenance of an effective safety management program (see also Required Characteristics GB.1.3.1.1.3 and GB.1.5 in the "Governing Body" chapter).*   1 2 3 4 5 NA

PL.1.2   The safety management program is based on monitoring and evaluation of organizational experience, applicable law and regulation, and accepted practice and includes*   1 2 3 4 5 NA

PL.1.2.1   policies and procedures for safety in all departments/services*;   1 2 3 4 5 NA

PL.1.2.2   a risk-assessment program that evaluates the impact of the buildings, grounds, equipment, occupants, and internal physical systems on patient care and safety*;   1 2 3 4 5 NA

PL.1.2.3   special attention to hazards related to the ages of the patients served*;   1 2 3 4 5 NA

PL.1.2.4   policies and procedures for the timely reporting and resolution of situations that pose an immediate threat to life, health, and/or property*;   1 2 3 4 5 NA

PL.1.2.4.1   The policies and procedures are approved in writing by the chief executive officer.*   1 2 3 4 5 NA

PL.1.2.5   The objectives, scope, organization, and effectiveness of the safety management program are evaluated at least annually and revised as necessary.*   1 2 3 4 5 NA

PL.1.3   A safety officer appointed by the chief executive officer or a designee and qualified by experience and/or education is responsible for the development, implementation, and monitoring of the safety management program.*   1 2 3 4 5 NA

Note: *For an explanation of the rating scale, see "Using the Manual," page ix.*

All asterisked items are key factors in the accreditation decision process. For an explanation of the use of key factors, see "Using the Manual," page ix.

PL.1.3.1 The safety officer manages an ongoing organizationwide process to collect and evaluate information about hazards and safety practices that is used to identify safety management issues; the information collection and evaluation system includes*   1 2 3 4 5 NA

PL.1.3.1.1 summaries of safety management, life safety management, equipment management, and utilities management deficiencies or problems, failures, user errors, and relevant published reports of hazards associated with any of these areas*;   1 2 3 4 5 NA

PL.1.3.1.2 documented surveys, performed at least semiannually, of all areas of the facility to identify environmental hazards and unsafe practices*;   1 2 3 4 5 NA

PL.1.3.1.3 a system for reporting and investigating all incidents that involve property damage, occupational illness, or patient, personnel, or visitor injury*; and   1 2 3 4 5 NA

PL.1.3.1.4 summaries of actions taken as a result of other organizationwide monitoring activities, including quality assessment and improvement.*   1 2 3 4 5 NA

PL.1.3.2 The safety officer analyzes identified safety management issues and develops recommendations for resolving them.*   1 2 3 4 5 NA

PL.1.3.3 The safety officer works with appropriate staff to implement recommendations and to monitor the effectiveness of the changes.*   1 2 3 4 5 NA

PL.1.3.3.1 The results of monitoring are reported to the safety officer.*   1 2 3 4 5 NA

PL.1.3.4 Summaries of identified issues are communicated at least annually to the governing body, chief executive officer, directors of all departments/services, and those responsible for other monitoring activities, including quality assessment and improvement.*   1 2 3 4 5 NA

PL.1.4 All new personnel are oriented to the safety management program, and all personnel participate in continuing safety education and training (see also Required Characteristic EA.1.2 in the "Educational Activities" chapter).*   1 2 3 4 5 NA

PL.1.4.1 The orientation and continuing education and training address general safety management issues, departmental safety plans, special hazards related to assigned duties, safety practices specific to the ages of the patients served, and changes in the safety management program.*   1 2 3 4 5 NA

PL.1.5 There is a hazardous materials and wastes program, designed and operated in accordance with applicable law and regulation, to identify and control hazardous materials and wastes; the program includes*   1 2 3 4 5 NA

PL.1.5.1 policies, procedures, and written criteria for identifying, handling, storing, using, and disposing of hazardous materials from receipt through use and hazardous wastes from generation to final disposal*;   1 2 3 4 5 NA

PL.1.5.2 training for and, as appropriate, monitoring of personnel who manage and/or regularly come into contact with hazardous materials and/or wastes*;   1 2 3 4 5 NA

All asterisked items are key factors in the accreditation decision process. For an explanation of the use of key factors, see "Using the Manual," page ix.

PL.1.5.3   monitoring of compliance with the program's requirements*; and

1 2 3 4 5 NA

PL.1.5.4   evaluation of the effectiveness of the program. As part of the organizationwide information collection and evaluation system (see Required Characteristic PL.1.3.1), a summary of the evaluation, including identified problems, failures, user errors, and relevant published information about environmental and occupational hazards, is reported to the safety officer.*

1 2 3 4 5 NA

PL.1.6   There is an emergency preparedness program designed to manage the consequences of natural disasters or other emergencies that disrupt the organization's ability to provide care and treatment; the program includes*

1 2 3 4 5 NA

PL.1.6.1   information about how the organization plans to implement specific procedures in response to environmental or man-made events*;

1 2 3 4 5 NA

PL.1.6.2   provisions for the management of space, supplies, communications, and security *;

1 2 3 4 5 NA

PL.1.6.3   provisions for the management of staff, including distribution and assignment of responsibilities and functions*;

1 2 3 4 5 NA

PL.1.6.4   provisions for the management of patients, including scheduling of services, control of patient information, and admission, transfer, and discharge*;

1 2 3 4 5 NA

PL.1.6.5   staff training in their roles during emergencies*; and

1 2 3 4 5 NA

PL.1.6.6   semiannual implementations of the plan, either in response to an emergency or in a planned drill.*

1 2 3 4 5 NA

PL.1.6.6.1   The organization's performance during implementations of the plan is evaluated, documented, and reported to the safety officer through the organizationwide information collection and evaluation system (see Required Characteristic PL.1.3.1).*

1 2 3 4 5 NA

STANDARD

PL.2   There is a life safety management program designed to protect patients, personnel, visitors, and property from fire and the products of combustion and to provide for the safe use of buildings and grounds.*

1 2 3 4 5 NA

REQUIRED CHARACTERISTICS

PL.2.1   Each building in which patients are housed overnight or receive treatment is in compliance with the appropriate provisions of the 1988 edition of the *Life Safety Code* ® of the National Fire Protection Association (NFPA), or equivalent protection is provided and documented.*†

1 2 3 4 5 NA

---

*The asterisked items are key factors in the accreditation decision process. For an explanation of the use of the key factors, see "Using the Manual," page ix.

†Effective January 1, 1989, the Joint Commission began referencing the NFPA 101®-1988, the Life Safety Code® (LSC) of the National Fire Protection Association. All facilities being surveyed will be evaluated using this edition of the LSC. Buildings for which plans were approved after January 1, 1989, will be evaluated as "new construction" under the applicable occupancy chapters of the LSC.

Life Safety Code® and NFPA 101® are registered trademarks of the National Fire Protection Association, Inc, Quincy, Massachusetts.

PL.2.1.1 When requirements of the *Life Safety Code* ® and these standards or their equivalents are not met, a comprehensive plan of correction is developed.*

1 2 3 4 5 NA

PL.2.1.2 When requirements for fire protection or environment and grounds safety are affected by construction, the organization institutes and documents interim life safety measures to temporarily compensate for the hazard posed by existing life safety deficiencies.*†

1 2 3 4 5 NA

PL.2.1.3 The interim life safety measures are continued and documented so that the level of life safety is not diminished in any occupied area and a safe environment is maintained throughout construction of or alteration to buildings or grounds.*†

1 2 3 4 5 NA

PL.2.2 There is an ongoing program designed to assure that the buildings and grounds are suitable to the nature of the services provided and the ages and other characteristics of the patient population served.*

1 2 3 4 5 NA

PL.2.2.1 New construction provides for the safe and convenient use of buildings and grounds by physically disabled individuals.*

1 2 3 4 5 NA

PL.2.2.2 The organization has specific policies for the maintenance, supervision, and safe use by patients of all grounds and equipment, including special activity areas.*

1 2 3 4 5 NA

PL.2.2.3 Emergency departments/services are readily identifiable and easily accessible.*

1 2 3 4 5 NA

PL.2.2.4 Compliance with the requirements of the program is documented.*

1 2 3 4 5 NA

PL.2.3 There is an ongoing program designed to establish and maintain fire safety.*

1 2 3 4 5 NA

PL.2.3.1 The program is established through the following*:

1 2 3 4 5 NA

PL.2.3.1.1 Procedures to identify and maintain all applicable required features of fire protection to *Life Safety Code* ® standards*;

1 2 3 4 5 NA

PL.2.3.1.2 Procedures for inspecting, testing, and maintaining fire-alarm and fire-detection systems, including quarterly testing of all circuits and annual preventive maintenance of all components*;

1 2 3 4 5 NA

PL.2.3.1.3 Procedures for inspecting and testing all automatic fire-extinguishing systems annually*;

1 2 3 4 5 NA

PL.2.3.1.4 Procedures for the management of portable fire extinguishers, including guidelines for their identification, placement, and use; a quarterly inspection program; and a regular maintenance program*; and

1 2 3 4 5 NA

PL.2.3.1.5 Procedures to review proposed acquisitions of bedding, window draperies and other curtains, furnishings, decorations, wastebaskets, and other equipment to identify issues related to fire safety.*

1 2 3 4 5 NA

PL.2.3.2 The program is maintained through the following:

All asterisked items are key factors in the accreditation decision process. For an explanation of the use of key factors, see "Using the Manual," page ix.

†*See Appendix D on page 75 for a listing of the Interim Life Safety Measures.*

PL.2.3.2.1   As appropriate to occupancy classification, a fire-alarm or fire-detection system that upon activation minimizes smoke transmission through control of designated fans and/or dampers in air-handling and smoke-management systems*;

PL.2.3.2.2   A fire plan that addresses appropriate staff response to a fire emergency and appropriate education and training for all personnel in all elements of the fire plan*;

1 2 3 4 5 NA

1 2 3 4 5 NA

PL.2.3.2.3   For all personnel on all shifts in all patient care buildings, quarterly conducting and evaluation of fire drills that test staff knowledge of the use and function of the fire-alarm systems, transmission of alarms, containment of smoke and fire, transfer to areas of refuge, fire extinguishment, assignment of specific duties, and preparation for building evacuation*; and

1 2 3 4 5 NA

PL.2.3.2.4   Dissemination and enforcement of an organizationwide smoking policy that discourages the use of smoking materials.*

1 2 3 4 5 NA

PL.2.3.2.4.1   Where smoking is permitted, there are appropriate policies to control the use of smoking materials.*

1 2 3 4 5 NA

PL.2.3.3   Compliance with the requirements of the program is documented.*

1 2 3 4 5 NA

PL.2.4   The life safety management program is used to identify and document *Life Safety Code*® and fire protection deficiencies, failures, and user errors that may threaten the patient care environment during a fire.*

1 2 3 4 5 NA

PL.2.4.1   When problems are identified, actions are taken to resolve them.*

1 2 3 4 5 NA

PL.2.4.1.1   The actions are documented.*

1 2 3 4 5 NA

PL.2.4.1.2   The actions are evaluated for effectiveness.*

1 2 3 4 5 NA

STANDARD

PL.3   There is an equipment management program designed to assess and control the clinical and physical risks of fixed and portable equipment used for the diagnosis, treatment, monitoring, and care of patients and of other fixed and portable electrically powered equipment.*

1 2 3 4 5 NA

REQUIRED CHARACTERISTICS

PL.3.1   Written criteria, which include characteristics of equipment function, clinical application, maintenance requirements, and equipment incident history, are used to identify equipment to be included in the program.*

1 2 3 4 5 NA

PL.3.1.1   Before a piece or type of equipment is used, it is evaluated for inclusion in the program, and the evaluation is documented.*

1 2 3 4 5 NA

PL.3.2   A current, accurate, unique inventory is kept of all equipment included in the program, regardless of the equipment's ownership or purpose.*

1 2 3 4 5 NA

---

*All asterisked items are key factors in the accreditation decision process. For an explanation of the use of key factors, see "Using the Manual," page ix.

PL.3.2.1   Each piece or type of equipment listed in the inventory has written equipment-testing procedures and user-training programs designed to manage the clinical and physical risks.*

1 2 3 4 5 NA

PL.3.2.1.1   Each piece of equipment is tested prior to initial use and at least annually thereafter; such testing is documented.*

1 2 3 4 5 NA

PL.3.2.1.2   Orientation and at least annual continuing education of individuals who use and/or maintain the equipment are documented.*

1 2 3 4 5 NA

PL.3.3   The equipment management program is used to identify and document equipment problems, failures, and user errors that have or may have an adverse effect on patient safety and/or the quality of care.*

1 2 3 4 5 NA

PL.3.3.1   When problems are identified, actions are taken to resolve them.*

1 2 3 4 5 NA

PL.3.3.1.1   The actions are documented.*

1 2 3 4 5 NA

PL.3.3.1.2   The actions are evaluated for effectiveness.*

1 2 3 4 5 NA

STANDARD

PL.4   There is a utilities management program designed to assure the operational reliability, assess the special risks, and respond to failures of utility systems that support the patient care environment.*

1 2 3 4 5 NA

REQUIRED CHARACTERISTICS

PL.4.1   Written criteria, which include utilities for life support, infection control, environmental support, and equipment support elements, are used to identify utilities to be included in the program.*

1 2 3 4 5 NA

PL.4.2   There is a reliable, adequate emergency power system to provide electricity to designated areas during interruption of the normal electrical source.*

1 2 3 4 5 NA

PL.4.2.1   As required by occupancy classification, the emergency power system provides electricity to at least the following:

PL.4.2.1.1   Alarm systems*;

1 2 3 4 5 NA

PL.4.2.1.2   Egress illumination*;

1 2 3 4 5 NA

PL.4.2.1.3   Elevators (at least one)*;

1 2 3 4 5 NA

PL.4.2.1.4   Emergency communication systems*; and

1 2 3 4 5 NA

PL.4.2.1.5   Illumination of exit signs.*

1 2 3 4 5 NA

PL.4.2.2   The emergency power system also provides electricity to the following areas, as applicable, based upon the services provided:

PL.4.2.2.1   Emergency care areas*;

1 2 3 4 5 NA

PL.4.2.2.2   Medical air compressors*;

1 2 3 4 5 NA

PL.4.2.2.3   Medical/surgical vacuum systems*;

1 2 3 4 5 NA

PL.4.2.2.4   Obstetric delivery rooms*;

1 2 3 4 5 NA

*All asterisked items are key factors in the accreditation decision process. For an explanation of the use of key factors, see "Using the Manual," page ix.

PL.4.2.2.5	Operating rooms*; and	1 2 3 4 5 NA
PL.4.2.2.6	Postoperative recovery rooms.*	1 2 3 4 5 NA

PL.4.3   A current, accurate, unique inventory is kept of all equipment for utility systems included in the program.*   1 2 3 4 5 NA

PL.4.4   Utility system operational plans are written to help assure reliability, control risks, reduce failures, and train users and operators of the systems.*   1 2 3 4 5 NA

PL.4.4.1   The organization develops procedures and establishes intervals for the testing and maintenance of equipment for utility systems included in the program.*   1 2 3 4 5 NA

PL.4.4.2   Tests and inspections that support operational reliability and manage risks are documented.*   1 2 3 4 5 NA

PL.4.4.3   Orientation and at least annual continuing education for individuals who use and/or maintain utility systems are documented.*   1 2 3 4 5 NA

PL.4.5   There is a current, complete set of documents that indicates the distribution of each utility system, including controls for a partial or complete shutdown.*   1 2 3 4 5 NA

PL.4.5.1   Where provided, emergency shutoff controls are labeled.*   1 2 3 4 5 NA

PL.4.6   The utilities management program is used to identify and document utility problems, failures, and user errors that are or may be a threat to the patient care environment.*   1 2 3 4 5 NA

PL.4.6.1   When problems are identified, actions are taken to resolve them.*   1 2 3 4 5 NA

PL.4.6.1.1   The actions are documented.*   1 2 3 4 5 NA

PL.4.6.1.2   The actions are evaluated for effectiveness.*   1 2 3 4 5 NA

COMMENTS AND RECOMMENDATIONS

Use this space to explain each 2, 3, 4, or 5 rating and to specify methods for better meeting the intent of the standard.

*All asterisked items are key factors in the accreditation decision process. For an explanation of the use of key factors, see "Using the Manual," page ix.

EDUCATIONAL ACTIVITIES

STANDARD

EA.1   The organization strives to improve the professional competence and skill, as well as the quality of performance, of the health care practitioners and other professional personnel it employs.   1 2 3 4 5 NA

REQUIRED CHARACTERISTICS

EA.1   The organization provides convenient access to a library(ies) that contains materials pertinent to the clinical, educational, administrative, and research services offered.   1 2 3 4 5 NA

EA.1.2   The organization provides adequate orientation and training to familiarize all personnel with its facilities and procedures.   1 2 3 4 5 NA

EA.1.3   The organization provides for personnel trained in cardiopulmonary resuscitation and in the use of emergency medical equipment to be in the facility during all hours of operation.*   1 2 3 4 5 NA

EA.1.4   The organization encourages participation in seminars, workshops, and other educational activities pertinent to its mission, goals, and objectives.   1 2 3 4 5 NA

EA.1.5   When attendance at educational activities is required of professional personnel, the organization accepts evidence of participation in relevant external educational programs.   1 2 3 4 5 NA

EA.1.6   Educational activities relate at least in part to the findings of quality assessment and improvement activities.   1 2 3 4 5 NA

EA.1.7   The organization provides a monitoring function designed to assure that educational resources available to its professional personnel are relevant to its mission, goals, and objectives.   1 2 3 4 5 NA

EA.1.8   The organization provides a monitoring function designed to verify the continued maintenance of licensure and/or certification of professional personnel.*   1 2 3 4 5 NA

COMMENTS AND RECOMMENDATIONS

Use this space to explain each 2, 3, 4, or 5 rating and to specify methods for better meeting the intent of the standard.

Note: *For an explanation of the rating scale, see "Using the Manual," page ix.*

The asterisked items are key factors in the accreditation decision process. For an explanation of the use of the key factors, see "Using the Manual," page ix.

SURGICAL AND ANESTHESIA SERVICES

This chapter applies to services for all patients who (1) receive general, spinal, or other major regional anesthesia or (2) undergo surgery or other invasive procedures when receiving general, spinal, or other major regional anesthesia and/or intravenous, intramuscular, or inhalation sedation/analgesia that, in the manner used in the organization, may result in the loss of the patient's protective reflexes. Examples of invasive procedures include, but are not limited to, percutaneous aspirations and biopsies, cardiac and vascular catheterizations, and endoscopies.

STANDARD

SA.1   When an organization provides surgical or anesthesia services, they are provided in a safe environment and are performed by qualified health care practitioners.*   1 2 3 4 5 NA

REQUIRED CHARACTERISTICS

SA.1.1   The organization limits the types of elective surgical or invasive procedures and anesthesia services performed in facilities it owns or operates to those procedures and services that are appropriate to its resources.*   1 2 3 4 5 NA

SA.1.1.1   The planned services are

SA.1.1.1.1   recommended by qualified professional personnel,   1 2 3 4 5 NA

SA.1.1.1.2   approved by the governing body,*   1 2 3 4 5 NA

SA.1.1.1.3   documented,   1 2 3 4 5 NA

SA.1.1.1.4   reviewed annually, and   1 2 3 4 5 NA

SA.1.1.1.5   revised as necessary.   1 2 3 4 5 NA

SA.1.1.2   Whenever the organization adds new services, they are reviewed for safety and effectiveness.   1 2 3 4 5 NA

SA.1.2   Responsibility for the direction of surgical services and that of anesthesia services provided by the organization is vested in physicians who are qualified to assume professional, organizational, and administrative responsibility for the quality of the respective services rendered.*   1 2 3 4 5 NA

Note: *For an explanation of the rating scale, see "Using the Manual," page ix.*

*The asterisked items are key factors in the accreditation decision process. For an explanation of the use of the key factors, see "Using the Manual," page ix.

SA. 1.3   Surgical procedures are performed only by licensed independent practitioners[†] who have been granted privileges to perform those procedures by the organization's governing body on the recommendation of qualified professional personnel and after professional review of the practitioners' documented education, training, experience, and competence.*   1 2 3 4 5 NA

SA. 1.4   Anesthesia care and surgical care provided to each patient are the responsibility of qualified licensed independent practitioners.*   1 2 3 4 5 NA

SA. 1.5   Qualified health care practitioners who provide surgical or anesthesia care have been granted privileges to provide such care by the governing body in accordance with Required Characteristics GB.1.6 through GB.1.6.2.2 in the "Governing Body" chapter of this *Manual.**   1 2 3 4 5 NA

SA. 1.6   The surgical and anesthesia services and care are provided under policies and procedures approved by the organization.*   1 2 3 4 5 NA

SA. 1.7   A sufficient number of nursing and other personnel are available to assist in the provision of surgical and anesthesia services.*   1 2 3 4 5 NA

       SA.1.7.1   Each individual providing such services is competent and appropriately supervised.*   1 2 3 4 5 NA

SA. 1.8   A registered nurse who is qualified by appropriate education, experience, and competence supervises nursing services.*   1 2 3 4 5 NA

SA. 1.9   The organization has a documented plan for transferring a patient to an appropriate hospital when hospitalization is indicated.*   1 2 3 4 5 NA

SA. 1.10   Procedures are established for obtaining blood, blood components, or blood products on a timely basis.*   1 2 3 4 5 NA

SA. 1.11   The history, physical examination, and preoperative studies are appropriate to the procedure and to the patient.*   1 2 3 4 5 NA

       SA.1.11.1   A policy is established that indicates the comprehensiveness of the history and physical examination and the specific studies that must be conducted for specific categories of surgical procedures or anesthesia.   1 2 3 4 5 NA

          SA.1.11.1.1   The policy specifies the time frame within which the history and physical examination are performed and/or updated prior to surgery or anesthesia.   1 2 3 4 5 NA

          SA.1.11.1.2   The physical examination is performed by a licensed independent practitioner who has appropriate clinical privileges.*   1 2 3 4 5 NA

       SA.1.11.2   Findings from the history and physical examination and specific studies are documented in the patient's medical record prior to surgery or anesthesia.*   1 2 3 4 5 NA

SA. 1.12   The informed consent of the patient or, if applicable, the patient's representative is obtained before anesthesia is administered and/or surgery is performed.*   1 2 3 4 5 NA

All asterisked items are key factors in the accreditation decision process. For an explanation of the use of key factors, see "Using the Manual," page ix.

[†]**licensed independent practitioner** *Any individual who is permitted by law and by the organization to provide patient care services without direction or supervision within the scope of the individual's license and in accordance with individually granted clinical privileges.*

SA.1.12.1   The consent is documented in the medical record.   1 2 3 4 5 NA

SA.1.13   Anesthesia care includes, but is not necessarily limited to, the following activities, which are documented in the medical record: 1 2 3 4 5 NA

SA.1.13.1   Preanesthesia evaluation*;   1 2 3 4 5 NA

SA.1.13.1.1   The preanesthesia evaluation includes a review of objective diagnostic data, the patient's history, and the results of the physical examination.   1 2 3 4 5 NA

SA.1.13.2   Determination by a licensed independent practitioner with appropriate clinical privileges that the patient is an appropriate candidate to undergo the planned anesthesia*;   1 2 3 4 5 NA

SA.1.13.3   Preparation of the patient*;   1 2 3 4 5 NA

SA.1.13.4   Reevaluation of the patient immediately prior to the induction of anesthesia*;   1 2 3 4 5 NA

SA.1.13.5   Appropriate monitoring of the patient during the administration of anesthesia*;   1 2 3 4 5 NA

SA.1.13.5.1   The dosage of all drugs and agents used is documented.*   1 2 3 4 5 NA

SA.1.13.6   Evaluation of the postoperative status of the patient and surveillance of the patient in an appropriately staffed and equipped recovery area.*   1 2 3 4 5 NA

SA.1.14   The procedure performed and the patient's status at the conclusion of surgery are immediately documented in the medical record for use in the recovery area.*   1 2 3 4 5 NA

SA.1.15   The complete findings of every procedure, the techniques used, and the condition of the patient following the procedure are written or dictated immediately after the procedure and authenticated by the individual who performed the procedure.*   1 2 3 4 5 NA

SA.1.15.1   This report is filed in the patient's medical record as soon as possible after surgery.*   1 2 3 4 5 NA

SA.1.16   With the exception of those tissues exempted by the governing body after medical review, tissues removed during surgery are examined by a pathologist.*   1 2 3 4 5 NA

SA.1.16.1   The pathologist's report of the examination is incorporated into the patient's medical record.*   1 2 3 4 5 NA

SA.1.17   A licensed independent practitioner who has appropriate clinical privileges and who is familiar with the patient is responsible for the decision to discharge the patient.*   1 2 3 4 5 NA

SA.1.17.1   When the responsible licensed independent practitioner is not present to make the decision to discharge or does not sign the discharge order,

SA.1.17.1.1   the name of the licensed independent practitioner responsible for the discharge is recorded in the patient's medical record*; and   1 2 3 4 5 NA

All asterisked items are key factors in the accreditation decision process. For an explanation of the use of key factors, see "Using the Manual," page ix.

SA.1.17.1.2 relevant discharge criteria are rigorously applied to determine the patient's readiness for discharge.*

1 2 3 4 5 NA

SA.1.17.1.2.1 The discharge criteria are approved by the licensed independent practitioner staff.*

1 2 3 4 5 NA

SA.1.17.2 Patients who have received anesthesia are discharged in the company of a responsible adult.*

1 2 3 4 5 NA

SA.1.18 A licensed independent practitioner qualified in resuscitative techniques is present or immediately available until all patients operated on each day have been evaluated and discharged.*

1 2 3 4 5 NA

SA.1.19 Each patient and his/her accompanying responsible adult are given instruction in follow-up care after surgery.*

1 2 3 4 5 NA

SA.1.19.1 The instructions include information on how to obtain appropriate help in the event of postoperative problems.*

1 2 3 4 5 NA

SA.1.19.2 The instructions are reviewed with the patient and his/her accompanying responsible adult.*

1 2 3 4 5 NA

SA.1.19.3 The instructions are given in writing to the patient and his/her accompanying responsible adult.*

1 2 3 4 5 NA

SA.1.20 The quality and appropriateness of surgical and anesthesia services are monitored and evaluated as part of the quality assessment and improvement program and in accordance with Required Characteristics QA.1.6.1 through QA.1.6.2.10.3 of the "Quality Assessment and Improvement" chapter in this *Manual.**

1 2 3 4 5 NA

SA.1.20.1 The monitoring and evaluation process includes a regular and systematic evaluation of patients who require hospitalization following surgery.*

1 2 3 4 5 NA

SA.1.20.2 The monitoring and evaluation process includes, but is not limited to, the collection and evaluation of objective data relating to morbidity and mortality.

1 2 3 4 5 NA

SA.1.21 A safe environment for treating surgical patients, including adequate safeguards to protect the patient from cross-infection, is provided.*

1 2 3 4 5 NA

SA.1.21.1 As evidence of a safe environment, at least the following requirements are met:

1 2 3 4 5 NA

SA.1.21.1.1 Appropriate space and equipment are provided.*

1 2 3 4 5 NA

SA.1.21.1.2 Each operating room is designed and equipped so that the types of surgery conducted can be performed in a manner that protects the health and well-being of all individuals in the area. (See the requirements of the National Fire Protection Association [NFPA 99-1987†] and applicable federal, state, and local regulations.)*

1 2 3 4 5 NA

SA.1.21.1.2.1 Appropriate ventilation and humidity control are provided in order to minimize the risk of infection and to provide for the safety of the patient.*

1 2 3 4 5 NA

---

*The asterisked items are key factors in the accreditation decision process. For an explanation of the use of the key factors, see "Using the Manual," page ix.

†NFPA 99, Standard for Health Care Facilities, © 1987.

SA.1.21.1.3   If inhalation anesthetic agents are present in an operating room, the room is constructed and equipped to meet the requirements of the NFPA. (See NFPA 99-1987[†] and applicable federal, state, and local fire codes.)*   1 2 3 4 5 NA

SA.1.21.1.4   Anesthetic apparatus is inspected and tested before each use by the practitioner who will administer the anesthetic.*   1 2 3 4 5 NA

SA.1.21.1.4.1   If found defective, the equipment is not used until the fault is repaired, and repair of the equipment is documented.*   1 2 3 4 5 NA

SA.1.21.1.5   Emergency power is available in operative and recovery areas.*   1 2 3 4 5 NA

SA.1.21.1.6   Suitable equipment and cleaning agents are provided for the regular cleaning of all interior surfaces.   1 2 3 4 5 NA

SA.1.21.1.7   Operating rooms are appropriately cleaned after each procedure.*   1 2 3 4 5 NA

SA.1.21.1.8   Suitable equipment is available for the rapid and routine sterilization of operating room materials.*   1 2 3 4 5 NA

SA.1.21.1.9   Sterilized materials are packaged and labeled in a consistent manner to maintain sterility and identify expiration dates.   1 2 3 4 5 NA

SA.1.21.1.10   A preventive maintenance schedule is established and maintained which includes periodic calibration, cleaning, and adjustment of all equipment, as appropriate.*   1 2 3 4 5 NA

SA.1.21.1.11   Provision is made for use of isolation precautions or, when indicated, for immediate transfer, when patients are known or suspected to have an infectious disease.*   1 2 3 4 5 NA

SA.1.21.1.12   Acceptable aseptic techniques are used by all individuals in surgical areas.*   1 2 3 4 5 NA

SA.1.21.1.13   Only authorized and properly attired personnel are allowed in surgical areas.*   1 2 3 4 5 NA

SA.1.21.1.14   Advanced cardiac life-support capabilities, including equipment, medication, and trained personnel, are in the facility whenever it is open to patients.*   1 2 3 4 5 NA

---

*The asterisked items are key factors in the accreditation decision process. For an explanation of the use of the key factors, see "Using the Manual," page ix.

[†]NFPA 99, Standard for Health Care Facilities, © 1987.

COMMENTS AND RECOMMENDATIONS

Use this space to explain each 2, 3, 4, or 5 rating and to specify methods for better meeting the intent of the standard.

PHARMACEUTICAL SERVICES

STANDARD

PS.1   Pharmaceutical services meet the needs of patients and are provided in accordance with professional practices and legal requirements.*   1 2 3 4 5 NA

REQUIRED CHARACTERISTICS

PS.1.1   Drugs and biologicals are stored, secured, prepared, dispensed, transported, administered, and discarded in compliance with applicable federal, state, and local laws.*   1 2 3 4 5 NA

PS.1.1.1   Written policies and procedures describe the mechanisms instituted to comply with applicable federal, state, and local laws.   1 2 3 4 5 NA

PS.1.1.2   Written policies specify the method for maintaining the integrity of emergency drug supplies regardless of location.   1 2 3 4 5 NA

PS.1.2   Records required to demonstrate that the organization dispenses drugs safely and complies with applicable federal, state, and local laws are maintained.*   1 2 3 4 5 NA

PS.1.2.1   Such records include, but need not be limited to, sufficiently detailed documentation of controlled drugs in order to provide for accurate reconciliation.   1 2 3 4 5 NA

PS.1.3   Pharmaceutical services the organization makes available through a contractual agreement are provided in accordance with the same professional practices and legal requirements that would be required if such services were provided directly by the organization.*   1 2 3 4 5 NA

PS.1.4   A pharmacy owned and operated by the organization is supervised by a licensed pharmacist.*   1 2 3 4 5 NA

PS.1.5   Patients are not required to use a pharmacy owned or operated by the organization.   1 2 3 4 5 NA

PS.1.6   The quality and appropriateness of medication usage are monitored and evaluated as part of the quality assessment and improvement program and in accordance with Required Characteristics QA.1.6.1 through QA.1.6.2.10.3 of the "Quality Assessment and Improvement" chapter in this *Manual.**   1 2 3 4 5 NA

Note: For an explanation of the rating scale, see "Using the Manual," page ix.

*The asterisked items are key factors in the accreditation decision process. For an explanation of the use of the key factors, see "Using the Manual," page ix.

COMMENTS AND RECOMMENDATIONS

Use this space to explain each 2, 3, 4, or 5 rating and to specify methods for better meeting the intent of the standard.

LABORATORY SERVICES AND PATHOLOGY

STANDARD

LP.1   Pathology and medical laboratory services provided or made available by the organization are designed to meet the needs of patients and are provided in accordance with professional practices and legal requirements.*   1 2 3 4 5 NA

REQUIRED CHARACTERISTICS

LP.1.1   Pathology and medical laboratory services provided or made available adequately support the organization's clinical capabilities.*   1 2 3 4 5 NA

LP.1.2   Pathology and medical laboratory services include, but need not be limited to, the following:

    LP.1.2.1 Conducting laboratory procedures that are appropriate to the needs of patients*;   1 2 3 4 5 NA

    LP.1.2.2 Performing tests in a timely manner*;   1 2 3 4 5 NA

    LP.1.2.3 Distributing test results within 24 hours after completion of a test*;   1 2 3 4 5 NA

        LP.1.2.3.1 A copy of the results is kept in the laboratory.*   1 2 3 4 5 NA

    LP.1.2.4 Performing and documenting appropriate quality control procedures.*   1 2 3 4 5 NA

        LP.1.2.4.1 Such procedures include, but need not be limited to,

            LP.1.2.4.1.1 calibrating equipment periodically* and   1 2 3 4 5 NA

            LP.1.2.4.1.2 validating test results through the use of standardized control specimens or laboratories.*   1 2 3 4 5 NA

LP.1.3   Authenticated, dated reports of all examinations performed are included in the patient's medical record.*   1 2 3 4 5 NA

LP.1.4   Pathology and medical laboratory services provided by the organization are directed by a pathologist or another physician who is qualified to assume professional, organizational, and administrative responsibility for the quality of services rendered.*   1 2 3 4 5 NA

LP.1.5   A sufficient number of competent, appropriately trained or educated, and supervised personnel are available to conduct laboratory work.*   1 2 3 4 5 NA

Note: *For an explanation of the rating scale, see "Using the Manual," page ix.*

*The asterisked items are key factors in the accreditation decision process. For an explanation of the use of the key factors, see "Using the Manual," page ix.

LP.1.6   Established procedures are followed in obtaining, identifying, storing, and transporting specimens.*   1 2 3 4 5 NA

LP.1.7   Complete descriptions of all test procedures performed in the laboratory, including sources of reagents, standards, and calibration procedures, are available.   1 2 3 4 5 NA

LP.1.7.1   Information concerning the basis for the listed "normal" ranges also is available.*   1 2 3 4 5 NA

LP.1.8   Space, equipment, and supplies sufficient for performing the volume of work with optimal accuracy, precision, efficiency, and safety are provided.   1 2 3 4 5 NA

COMMENTS AND RECOMMENDATIONS

Use this space to explain each 2, 3, 4, or 5 rating and to specify methods for better meeting the intent of the standard.

*All asterisked items are key factors in the accreditation decision process. For an explanation of the use of key factors, see "Using the Manual," page ix.

RADIOLOGY SERVICES

STANDARD

RS.1 Radiology services provided or made available by the organization are designed to meet the needs of patients and are provided in accordance with professional practices and legal requirements.*   1 2 3 4 5 NA

REQUIRED CHARACTERISTICS

RS.1.1 Radiology services provided or made available adequately support the clinical capabilities of the organization.*   1 2 3 4 5 NA

RS.1.2 Radiology services include, but need not be limited to, the following:

RS.1.2.1 Providing radiographic or fluoroscopic diagnostic and treatment services that are appropriate to the organization's function*;   1 2 3 4 5 NA

RS.1.2.2 Interpreting x-ray films and other radiographs and supplying reports in a timely manner*;   1 2 3 4 5 NA

RS.1.2.3 Providing in a timely manner summaries of radiotherapy performed*; and   1 2 3 4 5 NA

RS.1.2.4 Maintaining duplicate reports of services and retaining film in the radiology department for a period that is in accordance with applicable laws and the policies of the organization.*   1 2 3 4 5 NA

RS.1.3 A radiologist authenticates reports for all examinations except those reports of specific procedures that may be authenticated by physicians or dentists who are not radiologists but who have been determined to be qualified to authenticate such reports and who have been granted privileges by the governing body to do so.*   1 2 3 4 5 NA

RS.1.3.1 Such privileges are granted in accordance with Required Characteristics GB.1.6 through GB.1.6.2.2 in the "Governing Body" chapter of this *Manual.**   1 2 3 4 5 NA

RS.1.4 Authenticated, dated reports of all examinations performed are included in the patient's medical record.*   1 2 3 4 5 NA

RS.1.5 Radiology services provided by the organization are directed by a physician who is qualified to assume professional, organizational, and administrative responsibility for the quality of services rendered.*   1 2 3 4 5 NA

RS.1.6 A sufficient number of competent, appropriately trained or educated, and supervised personnel are available to conduct radiology services.*   1 2 3 4 5 NA

Note: *For an explanation of the rating scale, see "Using the Manual," page ix.*

**The asterisked items are key factors in the accreditation decision process. For an explanation of the use of the key factors, see "Using the Manual," page ix.*

RS.1.7   Policies and procedures address the safety and quality aspects of radiology services.*   1 2 3 4 5 NA

RS.1.7.1   These policies and procedures include, but need not be limited to, the following:

RS.1.7.1.1   Performing radiology services only on the written order of a physician, a dentist, or, to the extent permitted by law, other persons authorized by the organization to engage in the direct treatment of patients,*   1 2 3 4 5 NA

RS.1.7.1.1.1   such orders being accompanied by a concise statement of the reason for the examination;   1 2 3 4 5 NA

RS.1.7.1.2   Limiting the use of any radioactive sources to physicians who have been granted privileges for such use on the basis of their training or education, experience, and competence*; and   1 2 3 4 5 NA

RS.1.7.1.3   Regulating the use, removal, handling, and storage of any radioactive material.*   1 2 3 4 5 NA

RS.1.8   Adequate space, equipment, and supplies are provided for performing the volume of work with optimal accuracy, precision, efficiency, and safety.*   1 2 3 4 5 NA

RS.1.8.1   Specific safety factors include, but need not be limited to,

RS.1.8.1.1   precautions against electrical, mechanical, and radiation hazards*;   1 2 3 4 5 NA

RS.1.8.1.2   proper shielding where radiation sources are used*;   1 2 3 4 5 NA

RS.1.8.1.3   acceptable monitoring devices for all personnel who might be exposed to radiation to be worn in any area with a radiation hazard*;   1 2 3 4 5 NA

RS.1.8.1.4   the maintenance of records on personnel exposed to radiation*;   1 2 3 4 5 NA

RS.1.8.1.5   instructions to personnel in safety precautions and in the handling of emergency radiation hazards*; and   1 2 3 4 5 NA

RS.1.8.1.6   the periodic evaluation, by qualified personnel, of radiation sources and of all safety measures followed—including calibration of equipment—in compliance with federal, state, and local laws and regulations.*   1 2 3 4 5 NA

---

*All asterisked items are key factors in the accreditation decision process. For an explanation of the use of key factors, see "Using the Manual," page ix.

COMMENTS AND RECOMMENDATIONS

Use this space to explain each 2, 3, 4 or 5 rating and to specify methods for better meeting the intent of the standard.

EMERGENCY SERVICES

This chapter applies only to an organization that represents itself in name or in advertising material as a place where emergency medical care is available to the public.

STANDARD

ES.1   When the organization represents itself as providing emergency medical care services in life-threatening, limb-threatening, or function-threatening conditions beyond the occasional emergency that occurs in the normal course of any clinical practice, the evaluation and initial treatment for a patient seeking care are properly conducted by qualified health care practitioners, and appropriate services are provided or arranged.*   1 2 3 4 5 NA

REQUIRED CHARACTERISTICS

ES.1.1   The organization has the capability of providing initial evaluation and support or stabilization of patients of all ages with life-threatening, limb-threatening, or function-threatening conditions.*   1 2 3 4 5 NA

ES.1.2   At a minimum, equipment, medication, and appropriately trained or educated personnel needed to treat life-threatening, limb-threatening, or function-threatening conditions are present for patients of all ages during all hours of operation.*   1 2 3 4 5 NA

ES.1.3   Appropriate diagnostic radiology and clinical laboratory services are immediately available during all hours of operation for use in life-threatening, limb-threatening, or function-threatening conditions.*   1 2 3 4 5 NA

ES.1.4   At least one physician who is experienced and competent in the provision of emergency care is immediately available to the facility during all hours of operation.*   1 2 3 4 5 NA

ES.1.5   A physician is responsible for the evaluation and management of patients seeking emergency care.*   1 2 3 4 5 NA

ES.1.5.1   Initial patient evaluations are conducted promptly.*   1 2 3 4 5 NA

ES.1.5.2   Trained personnel may use guidelines established by staff physicians to determine the priority in which patients seeking care will be seen.   1 2 3 4 5 NA

Note: *For an explanation of the rating scale, see "Using the Manual," page ix.*

The asterisked items are key factors in the accreditation decision process. For an explanation of the use of the key factors, see "Using the Manual," page ix.

ES.1.6   A registered nurse qualified by appropriate training or education, experience, and competence in emergency care supervises nursing services.*

1 2 3 4 5 NA

ES.1.7   Nursing services are provided by a sufficient number of competent, appropriately trained or educated, and supervised personnel who are available for the volume and type of emergency services provided.*

1 2 3 4 5 NA

ES.1.8   The name of each patient who seeks care and his or her disposition at discharge are documented in a log.

1 2 3 4 5 NA

ES.1.9   When definitive care is required, there is a written plan for the transfer of a patient and pertinent patient care documents.*

1 2 3 4 5 NA

ES.1.9.1   This plan is in accordance with the local emergency medical system, when one exists.*

1 2 3 4 5 NA

ES.1.10   To facilitate continuity of care, a current list of appropriate professionals and referral and consultation services is available and used.*

1 2 3 4 5 NA

ES.1.10.1   Efforts are made to arrange appropriate follow-up care through the patient's primary care physician.*

1 2 3 4 5 NA

ES.1.11   Policies and procedures define the scope and conduct of treatment provided.*

1 2 3 4 5 NA

ES.1.11.1   These policies and procedures address differences in treatment due to patient age.

1 2 3 4 5 NA

ES.1.11.2   These policies and procedures address the management of specific types of emergencies.

1 2 3 4 5 NA

ES.1.12   The quality and appropriateness of emergency services provided are evaluated as part of the quality assessment and improvement program and in accordance with Required Characteristics QA.1.6.1 through QA.1.6.2.10.3 of the "Quality Assessment and Improvement" chapter of this *Manual.**

1 2 3 4 5 NA

ES.1.13   The organization is integrated into the local emergency medical system, when one exists.*

1 2 3 4 5 NA

ES.1.14   The organization provides information to the public that details the capabilities of the facility.*

1 2 3 4 5 NA

ES.1.15   Emergency services are available in the facility seven days per week, 24 hours per day.*

1 2 3 4 5 NA

All asterisked items are key factors in the accreditation decision process. For an explanation of the use of key factors, see "Using the Manual," page ix.

COMMENTS AND RECOMMENDATIONS

Use this space to explain each 2, 3, 4, or 5 rating and to specify methods for better meeting the intent of the standard.

INFIRMARY

This chapter applies to any unit of an ambulatory care organization that provides overnight accommodations of limited duration for patients who are being treated for noncritical illnesses, are recovering from surgery, or require observation, and who do not require all the skills and equipment of an acute care hospital.

STANDARD

IN.1   When infirmary care is provided, appropriate services are rendered within the defined capabilities of the organization.*   1 2 3 4 5 NA

REQUIRED CHARACTERISTICS

IN.1.1   There is a policy that defines the limitations of the scope of care provided in the unit.*   1 2 3 4 5 NA

IN.1.1.1   The policy includes clinical criteria for determining the eligibility of individuals for admission.   1 2 3 4 5 NA

IN.1.2   There is a written plan for the evaluation, admission, and discharge of patients.*   1 2 3 4 5 NA

IN.1.2.1   The plan designates which individuals are qualified to provide care or services in the unit.*   1 2 3 4 5 NA

IN.1.2.2   The plan designates who is responsible for the care or services patients receive.*   1 2 3 4 5 NA

IN.1.3   A physician with appropriate privileges is responsible for the medical care of each patient.*   1 2 3 4 5 NA

IN.1.3.1   Such privileges are granted in accordance with Required Characteristics GB.1.6 through GB.1.6.2.2 in the "Governing Body" chapter of this *Manual*.*   1 2 3 4 5 NA

IN.1.4   At least one registered nurse qualified by appropriate training or education, experience, and competence is on duty on each shift when patients are in the unit.*   1 2 3 4 5 NA

IN.1.5   There is a written plan for providing emergency services for patients in the unit.*   1 2 3 4 5 NA

IN.1.5.1   The plan includes the provision that a physician is on call 24 hours per day.*   1 2 3 4 5 NA

Note: For an explanation of the rating scale, see "Using the Manual," page ix.

*The asterisked items are key factors in the accreditation decision process. For an explanation of the use of the key factors, see "Using the Manual," page ix.

IN.1.5.2   The plan describes the procedures to be followed when a patient needs to be transferred to a nearby hospital.*

1 2 3 4 5 NA

IN.1.6   A patient's medical record contains information on each admission, including

IN.1.6.1   a current history and physical examination,*

1 2 3 4 5 NA

IN.1.6.2   diagnosis,*

1 2 3 4 5 NA

IN.1.6.3   treatment orders,*

1 2 3 4 5 NA

IN.1.6.4   physician notes,*

1 2 3 4 5 NA

IN.1.6.5   nursing notes,*

1 2 3 4 5 NA

IN.1.6.6   therapies administered,*

1 2 3 4 5 NA

IN.1.6.7   results of diagnostic studies,*

1 2 3 4 5 NA

IN.1.6.8   disposition,* and

1 2 3 4 5 NA

IN.1.6.9   follow-up instructions to patients.*

1 2 3 4 5 NA

IN.1.7   When any patient is admitted with a suspected or diagnosed communicable disease, appropriate isolation procedures are followed.*

1 2 3 4 5 NA

IN.1.8   The dietary needs of patients are met.

1 2 3 4 5 NA

IN.1.9   The quality and appropriateness of care are monitored and evaluated as part of the organization's quality assessment and improvement program and in accordance with Required Characteristics QA.1.6.1 through QA.1.6.2.10.3 of the "Quality Assessment and Improvement" chapter of this *Manual.**

1 2 3 4 5 NA

COMMENTS AND RECOMMENDATIONS

Use this space to explain each 2, 3, 4, or 5 rating and to specify methods for better meeting the intent of the standard.

*All asterisked items are key factors in the accreditation decision process. For an explanation of the use of key factors, see "Using the Manual," page ix.

TEACHING AND PUBLICATION ACTIVITIES

STANDARD

TP.1   The governing body has policies concerning teaching and publication activities of staff members and such policies are consistent with the organization's mission, goals, and objectives.   1 2 3 4 5 NA

REQUIRED CHARACTERISTICS

TP.1.1   Policies concerning teaching activities address the

TP.1.1.1   terms and conditions of reimbursement or other compensation;   1 2 3 4 5 NA

TP.1.1.2   reasonableness of the amount of time spent away from direct patient care and administrative activities; and   1 2 3 4 5 NA

TP.1.1.3   training of all students and postgraduate trainees, including the extent of their involvement in patient care activities.*   1 2 3 4 5 NA

TP.1.2   The policy concerning the provision of health care by personnel in any student or postgraduate trainee status provides for close and adequate supervision and for informing the patient of the status of the provider.*   1 2 3 4 5 NA

TP.1.3   Policies concerning publishing activities address the

TP.1.3.1   need for governing body approval when the views, policies, and procedures expressed in a publication are attributed to the organization;   1 2 3 4 5 NA

TP.1.3.2   terms and conditions of compensation from publication; and   1 2 3 4 5 NA

TP.1.3.3   cost of publication.   1 2 3 4 5 NA

COMMENTS AND RECOMMENDATIONS
Use this space to explain each 2, 3, 4, or 5 rating and to specify methods for better meeting the intent of the standard.

Note: *For an explanation of the rating scale, see "Using the Manual," page ix.*

*The asterisked items are key factors in the accreditation decision process. For an explanation of the use of the key factors, see "Using the Manual," page ix.

RESEARCH ACTIVITIES

STANDARD

RA.1   The organization establishes and implements policies concerning any research activities in which it is involved.   1 2 3 4 5 NA

REQUIRED CHARACTERISTICS

RA.1.1   Research activities are performed in accordance with professional practices and legal requirements.   1 2 3 4 5 NA

        RA.1.1.1   Research activities are monitored periodically.   1 2 3 4 5 NA

RA.1.2   Protocols for conducting research are approved by the governing body or its designee after medical and legal review.*   1 2 3 4 5 NA

RA.1.3   Any research activities carried out within the organization are appropriate to the expertise of staff and the resources of the organization.*   1 2 3 4 5 NA

RA.1.4   Individuals engaged in research are provided with adequate facilities.   1 2 3 4 5 NA

RA.1.5   Rights and welfare of every research subject are adequately protected.*   1 2 3 4 5 NA

        RA.1.5.1   The informed consent of the subject, in the language spoken by the subject, is obtained through adequate and appropriate methods.*   1 2 3 4 5 NA

COMMENTS AND RECOMMENDATIONS

Use this space to explain each 2, 3, 4, or 5 rating and to specify methods for better meeting the intent of the standard.

Note: *For an explanation of the rating scale, see "Using the Manual," page ix.*

The asterisked items are key factors in the accreditation decision process. For an explanation of the use of the key factors, see "Using the Manual," page ix.

APPENDIX A
REVISIONS SINCE THE 1990 EDITION

This appendix describes revisions approved by the Joint Commission Board of Commissioners for publication in the 1992 edition of the *Accreditation Manual for Ambulatory Health Care, Volume I.* If the Board approves any changes to this edition subsequent to publication of this *Manual*, the changes will be reported in *Joint Commission Perspectives*, the official newsletter of the Joint Commission. A complimentary copy of this newsletter is sent to each ambulatory health care organization accredited through the Joint Commission's Ambulatory Care Accreditation Services.

New glossary entries and changes to "General Administrative Policies and Procedures" and "Accreditation and Appeal Procedures" (Appendix B) are not discussed in this appendix.

QUALITY ASSESSMENT AND IMPROVEMENT

Both the preamble and those standards addressing monitoring and evaluation requirements have been modified to facilitate the transition from quality assurance to continuous quality improvement. The revisions are meant to shift the emphases of quality assessment and improvement activities away from an approach that is (1) program and discipline specific, (2) direct care focused, and (3) individual and problem oriented to one that encourages continuous improvement.

QA.1.6 through QA.1.6.2.10.3 These required characteristics were revised to clarify the steps in the monitoring and evaluation process. The identification of important aspects of patient care, the definition of indicators and usable data, and the methods for evaluating and using data have been expanded and clarified. Approved by the Board of Commissioners January 10, 1992; effective for accreditation purposes July 1, 1992.

SUMMARY LIST REQUIREMENTS

MEDICAL RECORDS

MR.1.9 through MR.1.9.3.4 These standards have been revised to clarify the purpose of the requirement, which is to facilitate continuity of care between multiple providers and, over time, for a single provider. The revised material parallels corresponding standards in the 1992 *Accreditation Manual for Hospitals, Volume I.* Approved by the Board of Commissioners January 10, 1992; effective for accreditation purposes July 1, 1992.

CARE OF THE TERMINALLY ILL PATIENT

On May 31, 1991, the Board of Commissioners approved standards addressing the care of terminally ill patients. These standards will be effective for accreditation purposes July 1, 1992.

RIGHTS AND RESPONSIBILITIES OF PATIENTS

RP.1.5.1 through RP.1.5.2.1* These required characteristics have been added to address advance planning for care and the patient's right of choice in treatment approaches.

QUALITY OF CARE

QC.1.1.10.1 This new required characteristic addresses the need for patient preferences regarding future treatment (that is, advance directives) to be communicated to other organizations to which the patient may be referred or transferred.

MEDICAL RECORDS

MR.1.2.1 This required characteristic has been added to assure that a patient's advance directives are included in the clinical information that is available to the health care staff.

PLANT, TECHNOLOGY, AND SAFETY MANAGEMENT

The "Plant, Technology, and Safety Management" chapter has been revised using standards that closely parallel corresponding standards previously incorporated in the *Accreditation Manual for Hospitals, Volume I* and the *Consolidated Standards Manual, Volume I.* Approved by the Board of Commissioners January 10, 1992; effective for accreditation purposes July 1, 1992.

---

*Standards in the "Rights and Responsibilities of Patients" chapter have been rearranged to follow a more logical progression.

APPENDIX B
ACCREDITATION AND APPEAL PROCEDURES

The Application for Survey and appropriate survey documents shall be completed by the organization seeking accreditation. After a survey has been conducted, the findings, survey documents, and any other relevant material or information received from any source shall be evaluated and acted upon as described in this appendix.

I.   Evaluation by Joint Commission Staff

A. *Review and Determination by Joint Commission Staff*

Joint Commission staff shall review survey findings, survey documents, and any other relevant material or information received from any source, and shall, in accordance with decision rules approved by the Accreditation Committee of the Board of Commissioners,

1. determine that the organization be accredited, with or without type I recommendations,* as described in paragraph VI of these procedures; or

2. determine to recommend to the Accreditation Committee that the organization be conditionally accredited; or

3. determine that the organization be conditionally accredited, if the organization does not challenge its survey findings in accordance with paragraph I.B; or

4. determine to recommend to the Accreditation Committee that the organization be denied accreditation; or

5. transmit a report of the staff's findings to the Accreditation Committee, with a recommendation to accredit the organization, with or without type I recommendations, as described in paragraph VI of these procedures; or

6. defer consideration while additional information regarding the organization's compliance status is reviewed by Joint Commission staff.

B. *Determination to Recommend Conditional Accreditation*

1. Notification to Organization of Areas of Noncompliance with Standards. If Joint Commission staff, based on survey findings, survey documents, and any other relevant material or information received from any source, determines to recommend that the organization be conditionally accredited, except in those circumstances described in Paragraph VI below, it will send the organization a copy of the draft accreditation report, outlining its findings and determination. The organization may

---

A type I recommendation is a recommendation or group of recommendations that determines, in part, the accreditation decision and that should receive the highest priority in the organization's plans for improvement. The organization's progress in complying with such recommendations will be monitored by the Joint Commission, at stated times during the accreditation cycle, through focused surveys, written progress reports, or both.

    a. accept the findings and determination of the staff, which will promptly result in a decision to conditionally accredit; or

    b. within 20 business days from receipt of the report, submit to the Joint Commission any documentation of its compliance with Joint Commission standards at the time of the survey that is not reflected in the draft accreditation report, along with an explanation of why such documentation was not available for review at the time of the survey; or

    c. request the Joint Commission to resurvey one or more of the areas that led to the recommendation of conditional accreditation. If the findings of the first survey are found to be valid, there will be no change in the recommendation, and the organization will be charged for the resurvey expense. If the findings of the survey result in a recommendation to accredit, the organization will not be charged for the resurvey expense.

2. Failure to Respond by the Organization. If, within 20 business days from receipt of the draft accreditation report, the organization does not submit to the Joint Commission any documentation of its compliance with Joint Commission standards at the time of the survey that is not reflected in the draft accreditation report, or request the Joint Commission to resurvey one or more of the areas that led to the recommendation of conditional accreditation, then the staff recommendation shall promptly result in a decision to conditionally accredit.

3. Consideration of the Organization's Response. Joint Commission staff shall review the organization's submission of additional information or resurvey findings, and shall, in accordance with decision rules approved by the Accreditation Committee,

    a. recommend to the Accreditation Committee that the organization be conditionally accredited; or

    b. recommend to the Accreditation Committee that the organization be denied accreditation; or

    c. determine that the organization be accredited, with or without type I recommendations, as described in paragraph VI of these procedures;or

    d. transmit a report of the staff's findings to the Accreditation Committee, with a recommendation to accredit the organization, with or without type I recommendations, as described in paragraph VI of these procedures.

C. *Determination to Recommend That Accreditation Be Denied*

1. Notification to Organization of Areas of Noncompliance with Standards. If Joint Commission staff, based on survey findings, survey documents, and any other relevant material or information received from any source, determines, in accordance with decision rules approved by the Accreditation Committee, to recommend to the Accreditation Committee that the organization be denied accreditation, except in those circumstances described in Paragraph VI below, it will send a copy of the draft accreditation report to the organization, outlining its findings and determination. The organization may

    a. accept the findings and determination of the staff; or

    b. within 20 business days from receipt of the report, submit to the Joint Commission any documentation of its compliance with Joint Commission standards at the time of the survey that is not reflected in the draft accreditation report, along with an explanation of why such documentation was not available for review at the time of the survey; or

c.   request the Joint Commission to resurvey one or more of the areas that led to the recommendation that accreditation be denied. If the findings of the first survey are found to be valid, there will be no change in the recommendation, and the organization will be charged for the resurvey expense. If the findings of the resurvey result in a recommendation to accredit or to conditionally accredit, the organization will not be charged for the resurvey expense.

2.   Failure to Respond by the Organization. If, within 20 business days from receipt of the draft accreditation report, the organization does not submit to the Joint Commission any documentation of its compliance with Joint Commission standards at the time of the survey that is not reflected in the draft accreditation report or request the Joint Commission to resurvey one or more of the areas that led to the recommendation that accreditation be denied, then Joint Commission staff shall recommend to the Accreditation Committee that the organization be denied accreditation.

3.   Consideration of the Organization's Response. Joint Commission staff shall review the organization's submission or resurvey findings, and shall, in accordance with decision rules approved by the Accreditation Committee,

a.   recommend to the Accreditation Committee that the organization be conditionally accredited; or

b.   recommend to the Accreditation Committee that the organization be denied accreditation; or

c.   determine that the organization be accredited, with or without type I recommendations, as described in paragraph VI of these procedures; or

d.   transmit a report of the staff's findings to the Accreditation Committee with a recommendation to accredit the organization, with or without recommendations, as described in paragraph VI of these procedures.

D. *Decisions by the President of the Joint Commission*

Anything outlined in paragraphs I.A.–I.C.3 of these procedures to the contrary notwithstanding, if the survey findings include mention of the existence of any condition that poses a threat to public or patient safety, the president of the Joint Commission, or if the president is not available, a vice-president of the Joint Commission designated by the president to do so, may promptly decide that the organization be denied accreditation. This action, and the findings that led to this action, shall be reported by telephone and in writing to the organization's chief executive officer and in writing to the authorities having jurisdiction. The president's decision shall be promptly reviewed by the Accreditation Committee in accordance with paragraph II of these procedures.

II.   **Review by the Accreditation Committee**

A. *Scope of Review*

The Accreditation Committee shall consider the decision of the president of the Joint Commission, or his/her designee, or the report and recommendation of the Joint Commission staff, and may review the survey findings, survey documents, any other relevant material or information received from any source, including any additional information supplied by the organization in response to this information, and the findings of any resurvey.

B. *Decision*

Following such consideration and review, the Accreditation Committee shall

1. accredit the organization, with or without type I recommendations, as described in paragraph VI of these procedures; or

2. conditionally accredit the organization; or

3. deny accreditation to the organization or confirm a decision by the president to deny accreditation; or

4. defer consideration while additional information regarding the organization's compliance status is gathered and reviewed by Joint Commission staff; or

5. order a resurvey or partial resurvey of the organization and an evaluation of the results, to the extent appropriate, by Joint Commission staff. Thereafter, Joint Commission staff shall transmit its report and recommendation to the Accreditation Committee for action, as provided in paragraph II.C of these procedures.

C. *Deferred Consideration*

Whenever the Accreditation Committee defers consideration pursuant to paragraph II.B.4 or II.B.5 of these procedures, Joint Commission staff shall review and report to the Accreditation Committee concerning the organization's compliance status. The Accreditation Committee may order any resurvey or partial resurvey necessary to determine such status.

Following such consideration and review, the Accreditation Committee shall

1. accredit the organization, with or without type I recommendations, as described in paragraph VI of these procedures; or

2. conditionally accredit the organization; or

3. deny accreditation to the organization; or

4. defer consideration while additional information regarding the organization's compliance status is reviewed by Joint Commission staff; or

5. order an additional resurvey or partial resurvey of the organization and an evaluation of the results, to the extent appropriate, by Joint Commission staff. Thereafter, Joint Commission staff shall transmit its report and recommendations to the Accreditation Committee for action, as provided in paragraph II.C of these procedures.

D. *Consultation and Education Alternative*

If the Accreditation Committee acts pursuant to paragraph II.B.3 or II.C.3 of these procedures to deny accreditation to the organization, and if the organization was not an accredited organization at any time during the two years before the survey, the Accreditation Committee may direct Joint Commission staff to inform the organization that, instead of requesting a hearing as provided in paragraph IV of these procedures, the organization may elect to consider the survey a consultation and education visit that does not result in an accreditation decision. An organization may elect the consultation and education option only once. Such an election shall be made in the same manner as a request for a hearing as provided in paragraph IV of these procedures. If such an election is made, the organization shall be eligible for resurvey without any waiting period. If the organization elects to be resurveyed, it shall be charged a new survey fee. The consultation and education alternative described in this paragraph does not apply in those instances in which the Accreditation Committee confirms a decision by the president of the Joint Commission, or his/her designee, pursuant to paragraph I.D of these procedures to deny accreditation.

III. Conditional Accreditation

A. *Plan of Correction*

An organization that is conditionally accredited by the Accreditation Committee, pursuant to paragraph II.B.2 or II.C.2 of these procedures, shall be required to submit a plan of correction within 30 business days of its receipt of notification of conditional accreditation. The plan shall outline the steps that will be taken by the organization to correct the deficiencies outlined in the accreditation decision report and the time periods in which the action will be taken.

B. *Joint Commission Staff Action*

Upon submission of the plan of correction by the organization, Joint Commission staff shall

1. if the plan of correction is not acceptable, notify the organization that it must submit a revised plan within 15 business days of receipt of the notification;

   a. if a second plan of correction, submitted pursuant to paragraph III.B.1, is not acceptable, recommend to the Accreditation Committee that the organization be denied accreditation; or

2. if the plan of correction is acceptable, notify the organization that a survey to determine the extent to which the deficiencies have been corrected will be conducted within approximately six months following the notification of approval of the plan, or sooner if the plan of correction indicates earlier resolution of deficiencies; or

3. if the organization fails to make the required submission of a plan of correction in response to either the first request or to the request for a revised plan of correction, recommend to the Accreditation Committee that the organization be denied accreditation.

C. *Survey to Determine Correction of Deficiencies*

Within approximately six months following Joint Commission staff's approval of the plan of correction, the Joint Commission shall conduct a survey of the organization to determine the degree to which deficiencies have been corrected.

D. *Review and Determination by Joint Commission Staff*

Joint Commission staff shall review the survey findings, survey documents, and any other relevant material or information received from any source. In accordance with decision rules approved by the Accreditation Committee, Joint Commission staff shall

1. recommend to the Accreditation Committee that the organization be accredited, with or without type I recommendations, as described in paragraph VI of these procedures; or

2. recommend to the Accreditation Committee that the organization be denied accreditation; or

3. defer consideration while additional information regarding the organization's compliance status is reviewed by Joint Commission staff. At the conclusion of this review, one of the recommendations outlined in paragraph III.D of these procedures shall be made to the Accreditation Committee.

E. *Action by the Accreditation Committee*

Following review of the recommendations of Joint Commission staff, the Accreditation Committee shall

1. accredit the organization, with or without type I recommendations, as described in paragraph VI of these procedures; or

2. deny accreditation to the organization; or

3. defer consideration while additional information regarding the organization's compliance status is reviewed by Joint Commission staff; or

4. order a resurvey or partial resurvey of the organization and an evaluation of the results, to the extent appropriate, by Joint Commission staff. Thereafter, Joint Commission staff shall transmit its report and recommendation to the Accreditation Committee for action, as provided in paragraph III.E of these procedures.

F. *Charges to the Organization*

The full costs of the conditional accreditation process shall be paid by the organization that receives conditional accreditation.

IV. Hearings

A. *Right to a Hearing*

An organization that has been denied accreditation pursuant to paragraph II.B.3, II.C.3, or III.E.2 of these procedures is entitled to a hearing before an Appeal Hearing Panel if the Joint Commission receives the organization's written request for the hearing within 20 business days after the organization receives the written notice of the Accreditation Committee's decision, including confirmation of a decision by the president, or his/her designee, to deny accreditation, as provided in paragraph IV.B of these procedures. An Appeal Hearing Panel shall be composed of at least three impartial individuals who are chosen by the president of the Joint Commission, or his/her designee. One member of the panel will be a member of the Board of Commissioners who did not participate in the accreditation decision.

B. *Notice of Right to a Hearing*

The Joint Commission shall promptly send the organization a written report of the Accreditation Committee's decision, the basis for the decision, the organization's right to a hearing, the dates of two scheduled Appeal Hearing Panels, and the time within which the organization must request, in writing, a hearing before one of those panels. Any request for a hearing may include a written statement of the organization's position.

C. *Notice of the Time and Place of a Hearing*

Any hearing to which an organization is entitled shall be held at the Joint Commission's central office except when the president of the Joint Commission, or his/her designee, determines otherwise for good cause shown. At least 20 calendar days before a hearing, the Joint Commission shall send the organization written notice of the time and place of the hearing and copies of any supplemental materials or information received from any source that the organization does not already have and that may affect any accreditation decision. The notice of the hearing shall advise the organization of the procedure to be followed at the hearing and, if feasible, of the identity and professional qualifications of the panel members.

D. *Continuance of a Hearing*

The president of the Joint Commission, or his/her designee, may continue the date of any hearing for good cause shown to the next scheduled Appeal Hearing Panel. An organization's request for such a continuance must be received by the Joint Commission in writing at least 15 calendar days before the scheduled date of the hearing.

E. *Procedure for the Conduct of a Hearing*

A hearing may be conducted with only two of the three panel members, provided one of them is the current member of the Board of Commissioners. Representatives of the organization may be accompanied by legal counsel, may make oral and written presentations, and may offer information at any hearing before an Appeal Hearing Panel. The organization may request the attendance of any Joint Commission field representative who participated in the survey and who is available to appear at the hearing. Such requests must be received within at least 15 calendar days before the hearing. Presentations or information concerning actions taken by the organization subsequent to the survey are not considered relevant to the validity of the original adverse decision.

F. *Adjournment of a Hearing*

After a hearing has commenced, an Appeal Hearing Panel may, if it chooses, suspend consideration for the purpose of receiving any additional information relating to the recommendation that it will make to the Board Appeal Review Committee. The panel may adjourn to another time or place, including reconvening by telephone conference, for this purpose.

G. *Report of Appeal Hearing Panel*

After a hearing has been completed, the Appeal Hearing Panel shall study the facts surrounding the original adverse decision and independently determine to recommend that the organization be accredited with or without type I recommendations, as described in paragraph VI of these procedures, or that the organization be conditionally accredited, or that accreditation be denied to the organization. The panel will submit a report of its findings, recommendations, and the rationale for its recommendations for consideration by the Board Appeal Review Committee. The Joint Commission shall send the organization written notice of the report of the Appeal Hearing Panel at least 30 calendar days before the meeting of the Board Appeal Review Committee at which the report will be considered. The notice shall inform the organization of the date of the meeting and of the organization's right to submit written responses or comments for consideration by the Board Appeal Review Committee. Any such written responses or comments must be received by the Joint Commision at least 15 calendar days before the meeting of the Board Appeal Review Committee.

V.   Review by the Board Appeal Review Committee

A. *Procedure for Review*

The report of an Appeal Hearing Panel shall be considered at the next regular meeting of the Board Appeal Review Committee. Two members will constitute a quorum. This meeting will generally be held by telephone conference, except when it is held in conjunction with meetings of the Board or other Board Committee(s). The Board Appeal Review Committee shall review the report of the Appeal Hearing Panel and any written responses or comments submitted by the organization pursuant to paragraph IV.E or IV.G of these procedures and shall take one of the following actions:

1. If the Appeal Hearing Panel recommends that the organization be accredited, the Committee shall

   a. accredit the organization, with or without type I recommendations, as described in paragraph VI of these procedures, after finding that there is substantial evidence to support the recommendation; or

   b. either deny accreditation to the organization or conditionally accredit the organization after finding that there is not substantial evidence to support the recommendation.

2. If the Appeal Hearing Panel recommends that the organization be conditionally accredited, the Committee shall

a. conditionally accredit the organization after finding that there is substantial evidence to support the recommendation; or

b. deny accreditation to the organization after finding that there is not substantial evidence to support the recommendation; or

c. make an independent evaluation of the report of the Appeal Hearing Panel and then decide to accredit the organization, with or without type I recommendations, as described in paragraph VI of these procedures.

3. If the Appeal Hearing Panel recommends that the organization be denied accreditation, the Committee shall

a. deny accreditation to the organization, after finding that there is substantial evidence to support the recommendation; or

b. make an independent evaluation of the report of the Appeal Hearing Panel and then decide to conditionally accredit or accredit the organization, with or without type I recommendations, as described in paragraph VI of these procedures.

The action taken by the Board Appeal Review Committee shall constitute the final accreditation decision of the Joint Commission.

B. *Participation*

No member of the Accreditation Committee or of the Appeal Hearing Panel who participated in an accreditation decision or recommendation concerning an organization, shall participate in any deliberations or vote of the Board Appeal Review Committee in its review of that accreditation decision or recommendation. This provision shall not preclude any Commissioner who participated in an appeal hearing as a member of the Appeal Hearing Panel from presenting and responding to questions about the report and recommendation of that Appeal Hearing Panel to the Board Appeal Review Committee.

VI. Procedure Relating to Type I Recommendations and Determination of Corrected Deficiencies

A decision of Joint Commission staff pursuant to paragraph I.A.1 or I.B.3.c, or I.C.3.c of these procedures, of the Accreditation Committee pursuant to paragraph II.B.1, II.C.1, or III.E.1 of these procedures, or of a Board Appeal Review Committee, as provided in paragraph V.A of these procedures, to accredit an organization may be made contingent upon satisfactory implementation of type I recommendations. The organization may be conditionally accredited or its accreditation may be withdrawn if it does not correct or document the correction of the specified deficiencies within the time specified in the notice of the decision to the organization. In such circumstances, the procedures for sending a draft notice and obtaining a response from the organization set out in Paragraphs I.B and I.C are not applicable. Joint Commission staff, through the use of surveys or partial surveys, or through other means, such as written progress reports, shall determine whether the organization has corrected the deficiencies within the time provided and shall report its findings to the organization. If Joint Commission staff determines that the organization has not corrected the deficiencies within the time provided, staff shall, as appropriate,

1. provide another opportunity to the organization to correct or document the correction of deficiencies, as provided in any applicable decision rules approved by the Accreditation Committee; or

2. recommend that the organization be placed into conditional accreditation status with a conditional follow-up visit in approximately four months; or

3. recommend to the Accreditation Committee that the organization be denied accreditation, if certain deficiencies, specified in decision rules approved by the Accreditation Committee, have not been corrected or the correction of which has not been documented after the specified number of opportunities given to the organization to do so.

VII. Final Accreditation Decision

A. The action taken by Joint Commission staff shall constitute the final decision of the Joint Commission to accredit the organization, when taken pursuant to paragraph I.A.1, I.B.3.c, or I.C.3.c of these procedures.

B. The action taken by the Accreditation Committee shall constitute the final decision of the Joint Commission to

1. accredit the organization, when taken pursuant to paragraph II.B.1, II.C.1, or III.E.1 of these procedures; or

2. conditionally accredit the organization, when taken pursuant to paragraph II.B.2 or II.C.2 of these procedures; or

3. deny accreditation to the organization, when taken pursuant to paragraph II.B.3, II.C.3, or III.E.2 of these procedures, and the organization neither requests a hearing pursuant to paragraph IV.A of these procedures nor elects to have the survey treated as a consultation and education visit, as provided in paragraph II.D of these procedures.

VIII. Status of the Organization Pending and After Appeal and Effective Date of a Final Decision

A. The accreditation status of an accredited organization shall continue in effect pending any final accreditation decision.

B. A final decision to accredit an organization shall be considered effective as of the first day after completion of the organization's survey from which the decision results.

C. A decision to deny accreditation to an organization shall become final and effective

1. as of the date of the decision when the decision is made by the Board Appeal Review Committee pursuant to paragraph V of these procedures; or

2. at the expiration of the time during which an organization may, but does not, request a hearing before an Appeal Hearing Panel, pursuant to paragraph IV.A of these procedures; or

3. on receipt by the Joint Commission, before a decision to deny accreditation to the organization by the Board Appeal Review Committee of written notification from the organization that it accepts the decision made by the Accreditation Committee, pursuant to paragraph II.B.3, II.C.3, or III.E.2 of these procedures and thereby withdraws its appeal.

IX. Notice

Any notice required by these accreditation procedures to be given to an organization shall be addressed to the organization at its post office address as shown in Joint Commission records and shall be sent to the organization by U.S. registered mail, return receipt requested, with postage prepaid. Any notice required to be given to the Joint Commission by the organization shall be sent by the organization in the same manner and shall be addressed to the Office of the Vice-President for Accreditation Surveys, Joint Commission on Accreditation of Healthcare Organizations, One Renaissance Boulevard, Oakbrook Terrace, Illinois 60181.

APPENDIX C
SURVEYOR MATERIALS

The materials on the following pages are for surveyor use only. They are included here to help ambulatory health care organizations perform self-assessments.

NOTE TO THE SURVEYOR: *At the Opening Conference, please provide the chief executive officer/executive director with this page of Appendix C. This form must be complete when returned to you prior to the CEO Exit Conference. This information will be used to update the files kept on the organization, and for purposes of sending the notification of the results of the survey to the appropriate persons.*

FACE SHEET/PROFILE INFORMATION

1. Organization name _____
   Street _____ Box # _____
   City _____ State _____ Zip _____

2. CEO/Executive director name _____
   Title _____ Telephone _____

3. Medical director name _____
   Title _____

4. (Applicable only when an additional letter and notification of accreditation survey results should be sent to the Governing Body/Board or a corporate/ owner office)
   Name _____ Title _____
   Address (if different from above) _____

5. Please circle owner code:

12 State	15 Joint ownership by city/county	47 IHS
13 County	16 Hospital district/authority	45 Veterans
14 City	21 Church operated, nonprofit	Administration
40 Coast Guard	23 Other, not for profit	48 Fed, Department
41 Air Force	31 Individual, for profit	of Justice
42 Army	33 Corporation, for profit	46 Fed, not delineated
43 Navy	44 U.S. Public Health (non-IHS)	above

6. Total number of physicians _____

7. Total number of personnel other than physicians _____

8. Total **annual** number of patient visits _____

9. Total number of locations providing health care services _____
   (Not applicable to managed care organizations)

SURVEY INFORMATION To be completed by the surveyor team

1. Locations surveyed

Name and location of provider site	Type of service	Annual visits/membership
_____	_____	_____
_____	_____	_____
_____	_____	_____
_____	_____	_____
_____	_____	_____

SURVEYOR INFORMATION

Please note that if there is more than one surveyor team—for example, when **multiple sites** are surveyed—**each chapter** completed *must* indicate the name of the managed care organization; the provider site name; the surveyor name; and the surveyor's ID number (the number on your surveyor ID badge). Thank you.

1. Surveyor Signature _____,MD ID# _____
   (please print name) _____

2. Surveyor Signature _____,Adm ID# _____
   (please print name) _____

COMMENTS

The survey team should describe any noteworthy or unique problems or characteristics that would provide background information relating to the survey. In addition, the team should provide its impressions of the overall status of the organization, which include a description of any significant changes since the last survey.

_____

_____

_____

_____

PUBLIC INFORMATION INTERVIEW REPORT

Organization _____ City and state _____
Date held _____ Report completed by _____

Please provide a brief description of the reason for this interview and any issues that relate to the survey process. Be certain to include the name(s) of all persons present at the interview.

_____

_____

_____

_____

APPENDIX D
INTERIM LIFE SAFETY MEASURES

Interim Life Safety Measures (ILSM) are a series of 11 administrative actions required to be taken to temporarily compensate for the hazards posed by existing *Life Safety Code* ® (*LSC*) deficiencies or construction activities.*

Implementation of ILSM is required in or adjacent to all construction areas and throughout buildings with existing *LSC* deficiencies. ILSM apply to all personnel, including construction workers, must be implemented upon project development, and continuously enforced through project completion.

ILSM are intended to provide a level of life safety comparable to that described in chapters 1 through 7, 31, and the applicable occupancy chapters of the 1988 edition of the *LSC* (*NFPA 101*). Each ILSM action must be documented. Except as stated below, frequencies for inspection, testing, training, and monitoring and evaluation must be established by the organization.

ILSM consist of the following actions:

a) Ensuring exits provide free and unobstructed egress. Personnel shall receive training if alternative exits must be designated.

b) Ensuring free and unobstructed access to emergency departments/services and for emergency forces.

c) Ensuring fire alarm, detection, and suppression systems are not impaired. A temporary, but equivalent, system shall be provided when any fire system is impaired. Temporary systems must be inspected and tested monthly.

d) Ensuring temporary construction partitions are smoke tight and built of noncombustible materials.

e) Providing additional fire fighting equipment and use training for personnel.

f) Prohibiting smoking in or adjacent to all construction areas.

g) Developing and enforcing storage, housekeeping, and debris removal policies and procedures that reduce the flammable and combustible fire load to the lowest level necessary for daily operations.

h) Conducting a minimum of two fire drills per shift per quarter.

i) Increasing hazard surveillance of buildings, grounds, and equipment with special attention to excavations, construction areas, construction storage, and field offices.

j) Training personnel when structural or compartmentation features of fire safety are compromised.

k) Conducting organizationwide safety education programs to ensure awareness of any *LSC* deficiencies, construction hazards, and these ILSM.

Note: If questions arise concerning the implementation and use of ILSM, contact the Department of Plant and Technology Management at the Joint Commission.

Life Safety Code® and NFPA 101® are registered trademarks of the National Fire Protection Association, Inc, Quincy, Massachusetts.

GLOSSARY

abusable supplies
Any medical items or equipment that should be used only by authorized personnel. These items may include, for example, needles, drugs, and prescription pads.

accreditation
A determination by the Joint Commission that an eligible organization complies substantially with applicable Joint Commission standards.

accreditation appeal
The process through which an organization that has been denied accreditation exercises its right to a hearing by an Appeals Hearing Panel followed by a review of the panel's report and recommendation by the Board of Commissioners.

Accreditation Committee
The committee of the Board of Commissioners responsible for oversight of the accreditation decision process.

accreditation cycle
The three-year term at the conclusion of which accreditation expires unless a full survey is performed.

accreditation decision
The conclusion reached regarding an organization's status after evaluation of the results of the on-site survey, recommendations of the surveyor(s), and any other relevant information, such as documentation of compliance with standards, documentation of plans to correct deficiencies, or evidence of recent improvements. The decision may be accreditation with commendation, accreditation, conditional accreditation, or not accredited.

> **accreditation with commendation** The highest accreditation decision, awarded to an organization that has demonstrated exemplary performance.
>
> **accreditation** See accreditation.
>
> **conditional accreditation** A determination that substantial standards compliance deficiencies exist in an organization. Findings of correction, which serve as the bases for further consideration of awarding full accreditation, must be demonstrated through a follow-up survey at six months.
>
> **not accredited** An accreditation decision that results when an organization has not been granted accreditation, when its accreditation is withdrawn by the Joint Commission, or when it withdraws from the accreditation process. This designation also describes any organization that has never applied for accreditation.

accreditation decision grid

A numerical summary of aggregated scores, reflecting levels of compliance, assigned to standards in the survey process. Each score on the grid reflects an assigned level of compliance for standards relating to a key performance area, such as infection control or safety management.

accreditation decision grid score

An aggregated score developed to reflect overall performance of the organization as reflected in the accreditation decision grid. Each performance area is weighted according to its importance, indicated by a Roman numeral (I = most important). The performance area score is multiplied by the weight to develop the percentage of a perfect score of 100% attained by the organization.

accreditation duration

The three-year time period during which an organization found to be in substantial compliance with Joint Commission standards is awarded accreditation. To maintain accreditation for a three-year period, satisfactory resolution of any identified issues is required.

accreditation history

An account of past accreditation decisions for an organization. The accreditation history may be publicly disclosed by the Joint Commission upon request.

accreditation survey

An evaluation of an organization to assess its level of compliance with applicable standards and make determination regarding its accreditation status. The survey includes evaluation of documentation of compliance provided by personnel; verbal information concerning the implementation of standards, or examples of their implementation, that will enable surveyors to make a determination of compliance; and surveyors' on-site observations. The survey also provides the opportunity for education and consultation to organizations regarding standards compliance.

> **focused survey** A survey conducted during the accreditation cycle to assess the degree to which an organization has improved its level of compliance relating to specific recommendations. The subject matter of the survey is confined to the area(s) of identified deficiency in compliance.

> **survey report** The report resulting from the on-site assessment of an organization outlining identified deficiencies in standards compliance. It also outlines the nature of the accreditation decision, including enumeration of type I recommendations, the implementation of which will be monitored by the Joint Commission through the conduct of focused surveys or requests for written progress reports. The supplement to the report may also include other recommendations (type II) that are designed to assist the organization in improving its performance.

> **survey team** The group of health care professionals who work together to perform an accreditation survey.

> **surveyor** A physician, a nurse, an administrator, a laboratorian, or any other health care professional who meets Joint Commission surveyor selection criteria, evaluates standards compliance, and provides education and consultation regarding standards compliance to surveyed organizations.

> **tailored survey** A survey where standards from more than one standards manual are used in assessing compliance; it may include using specialist surveyors appropriate to the standards selected for survey. See standards manuals.

aspects of care, important
Care activities or processes that occur frequently or affect large numbers of patients; that place patients at risk of serious consequences if not provided correctly, if incorrect care is provided, or if correct care is not provided; and/or that tend to produce problems for patients or staff. Such activities or processes are deemed most important for purposes of monitoring and evaluation.

authenticate
To prove authorship, for example, by written signature, identifiable initials, or computer key.

biologicals
Medicines made from living organisms and their products including serums, vaccines, antigens, and antitoxins.

Board of Commissioners
The governing body of the Joint Commission.

bylaws
A governance framework that establishes the roles and responsibilities of a body and its members.

cardiopulmonary resuscitation (CPR)
The administration of artificial heart and lung action in the event of cardiac and/or respiratory arrest. The two major components of cardiopulmonary resuscitation are artificial ventilation and closed-chest cardiac massage.

chief executive officer (CEO)
The individual appointed by the governing body to act on its behalf in the overall management of the organization. Other job titles for this position include administrator, superintendent, director, executive director, president, vice-president, and executive vice-president.

chief executive officer exit conference
The meeting involving the surveyor(s), the chief executive officer, the chair of the governing body, the director of nursing, the medical director, and others, which is held at the conclusion of an on-site accreditation survey. The purpose of this meeting is for the surveyor(s) to present any findings of significant standards compliance problems and the potential impact of these on the final accreditation decision, and to provide the opportunity for conference participants to clarify issues.

clinical privileges
Authorization granted by the governing body to a practitioner to provide specific patient care services in the organization, within defined limits, based on an individual practitioner's license, education, training, experience, competence, health status, and judgment.

> **delineation of clinical privileges** The process of listing the specific clinical privileges an organization's staff member may be granted.

competence/competency
Capacity equal to requirement, as in "the competence of a medical or professional staff member."

compliance
To act in accordance with, as in "compliance with a standard."

compliance level A measure of the extent to which an organization acts in accordance with a specified standard, including

substantial compliance An organization consistently meets all major provisions of a specified standard; designated by a score 1.

significant compliance An organization meets most provisions of a standard; designated by a score 2.

partial compliance An organization meets some provisions of a standard; designated by a score 3.

minimal compliance An organization meets few provisions of a standard; designated by a score 4.

noncompliance An organization fails to meet the provisions of a standard; designated by a score 5.

not applicable The standard does not apply to the organization; designated by NA.

confidentiality and disclosure policy

A policy, overseen by the Executive Committee of the Board of Commissioners of the Joint Commission, governing the following:

(1) the confidentiality of certain organization information, including that obtained before, during, or following the accreditation survey; all materials that may contribute to the accreditation decision; standards compliance recommendations; and written staff analyses and Accreditation Committee minutes and agenda materials; and

(2) the disclosure of certain organization information, including that subject to public release; aggregate standards compliance data; and information subject to release to designated government agencies under specified circumstances.

confidentiality as a patient right

A patient's right, within the law, to personal and informational privacy, including his/her patient record.

continuing education

Education beyond initial professional preparation that is relevant to the type of patient care delivered in the organization, that provides current knowledge relevant to an individual's field of practice, and that is related to findings from quality assessment and improvement activities.

continuity of care

A component of patient care quality consisting of the degree to which the care needed by a patient is coordinated among practitioners and across organizations and time.

criteria

Expected level(s) of achievement against which performance or care can be evaluated.

criteria for survey eligibility Conditions necessary for organizations to be surveyed for accreditation. The criteria address the structure, functions, and services of the organization.

contract

A formal agreement with any organization, agency, or individual that specifies the services, personnel, products, and/or space provided by, to, or on behalf of the organization and specifies the consideration to be expended in exchange. The agreement is approved by the governing body.

data

The collection of material or facts on which a discussion or an inference is based, such as indicator data used to identify processes or outcomes that may be improved.

delineation of clinical privileges

See clinical privileges.

dentist

An individual who has received the degree of either doctor of dental surgery or doctor of dental medicine and who is licensed to practice dentistry.

diagnosis

A scientifically or medically acceptable term given to a complex of symptoms (disturbances of function or sensation of which the patient is aware), signs (disturbances that the physician or another individual can detect), and findings (detected by laboratory, x-ray, or other diagnostic procedures, or responses to therapy).

diagnostic radiology services

The delivery of care pertaining to the use of radiant energy for the diagnosis of disease. Standards are applied to evaluate an organization's performance in providing diagnostic radiology care.

> **medical radiation physicist, qualified** An individual who is certified by the American Board of Radiology in the appropriate disciplines of radiologic physics, including diagnostic, therapeutic, and/or medical nuclear physics; or an individual who demonstrates equivalent competency in these disciplines.

> **radiologic technologist, qualified** An individual who is a graduate of a program in radiologic technology approved by the Council on Medical Education of the American Medical Association or who has the documented equivalent in education and training.

documentation

The process of recording information in the medical record and other source documents.

> **quality of documentation** The degree to which information recorded in source documents is accurate and complete, and is performed in a timely manner.

drug

Any chemical compound that may be used on or administered to patients/residents as an aid in the diagnosis, treatment, or prevention of disease or other abnormal condition.

> **drug administration** The act in which a prescribed dose of an identified drug is given to a patient.

> **drug allergies** A state of hypersensitivity induced by exposure to a particular drug antigen resulting in harmful immunologic reactions on subsequent drug exposures, such as penicillin drug allergy.

> **drug dispensing** The issuance of one or more doses of a prescribed medication by a pharmacist or other authorized person to another person responsible for administering it.

emergency preparedness plan/program

A component of an organization's safety management program designed to manage the consequences of natural disasters or other emergencies that disrupt the organization's ability to provide care and treatment.

emergency services

An organization that represents itself in name or in advertising material as a place where emergency medical care is available to the public.

evaluation

A determination of worth or an appraisal, as in "the evaluation of a facility's performance."

focused survey

See accreditation survey.

governing body

The individual(s), group, or agency that has ultimate authority and responsibility for establishing policy, maintaining quality patient care, and providing for organizational management and planning. Standards are applied to evaluate the performance of an organization's governing body.

> **governing body bylaws** Rules that establish the roles and responsibilities of the governing body.

guideline, scoring

Descriptive tool that is used to assist hospitals in their efforts to comply with Joint Commission standards and to determine degrees of compliance. Scoring guidelines are described in the *Accreditation Manual for Ambulatory Health Care, Volume II.*

hazardous area

Any space with contents that, because of their basic nature (as in the case of flammable liquids) or because of the quantity of combustible materials involved, represent a significantly higher hazard than would otherwise be typical of a facility. Consult the 1988 edition of the *Life Safety Code* ® (NFPA 101®) for further information.

health care (or healthcare) organization

A generic term used to describe many types of organizations that provide health care services.

indicator

Measurement tool used to monitor the quality of important governance, management, clinical, and support functions and processes of a health care organization.

infirmary

A unit of an ambulatory health care organization that provides overnight accommodations of limited duration for patients who are being treated for noncritical illnesses, are recovering from surgery, or require observation and who do not require all the skills and equipment of an acute care hospital.

intent of standard

A brief explanation of the meaning and significance of a standard.

invasive procedure

A procedure involving puncture or incision of the skin or insertion of an instrument or foreign material into the body, including, but not limited to, percutaneous aspirations and biopsies, cardiac and vascular catheterizations, endoscopies, reconstructions, angioplasties, and implantations, and excluding venipuncture and intravenous therapy.

Joint Commission on Accreditation of Healthcare Organizations (JCAHO)

An independent, not-for-profit organization dedicated to improving the quality of care in organized health care settings. Founded in 1951, its members are the American College of Physicians, the American College of Surgeons, the American Dental Association, the American Hospital Association, and the American Medical Association. The major functions of the Joint Commission include organizational standards development, award of accreditation decisions, and provision of education and consultation to health care organizations.

leaders, organization

The group of individuals that set expectations, develop plans, and implement procedures to assess and improve the quality of the organization's governance, management, clinical, and support functions and processes. Leaders include at least the leaders of the governing body; the chief executive officer and other senior managers; the elected and/or appointed leaders of the medical staff and the clinical departments and other medical staff members in organization administrative positions; the director of nursing and other senior nursing leaders; and other key leaders.

leadership interview

A meeting of all surveyors present on the first day of the survey with the senior leadership of the organization for the purpose of making an assessment of how the organization's leaders work together in quality improvement activities, the roles that each of the major components of the organization play in its management, and the extent to which the organization is meeting the standards requirements for communication and cooperation.

licensed independent practitioner

Any individual who is permitted by law and by the organization to provide patient care services without direction or supervision, within the scope of the individual's license and in accordance with individually granted clinical privileges.

Life Safety Code ®

A set of standards compiled and published by the National Fire Protection Association and referenced by the Joint Commission to evaluate health care organizations under its life safety management program.

life safety management program

A component of an organization's plant, technology, and safety management program designed to protect patients/residents, personnel, visitors, and property from fire and the products of combustion and to provide for the safe use of buildings and grounds.

medical history

A component of the medical record consisting of an account of a patient's history, obtained whenever possible from the patient; it includes at the least the following information: chief complaint, details of the present illness, relevant past history, and a relevant inventory by body systems.

medical record

The account compiled by health care professionals of patients' medical history, present illness, findings on examination, details of treatment, and notes on progress. The medical record is the legal record of care.

medical record, complete

A medical record is complete when (1) its contents reflect the diagnosis, results of diagnostic tests, therapy rendered, condition and in-hospital progress of the patient, and condition of the patient at discharge; and (2) its contents, including any required clinical resume or final progress notes, are assembled and authenticated, and all final diagnoses and any complications are recorded without the use of symbols or abbreviations.

medical record practitioner, qualified

An individual who is eligible for certification as a registered record administrator (RRA) or as an accredited record technician (ART) by the American Medical Record Association, or who is a graduate of a school of medical record science accredited jointly by the Committee on Allied Health Education and Accreditation (CAHEA) and the American Medical Record Association; or an individual who has the documented equivalent education, training, and/or experience.

medical record services

The activities designed to ensure the accuracy, completeness, timeliness, accessibility, and safe, secure, and confidential storage of patients' medical records. Standards are applied to evaluate an organization's performance in providing medical record services.

medication

Any substance, whether a prescription or over-the-counter drug, that is taken orally or injected, inserted, topically applied, or otherwise administered to a patient.

mission statement

A written expression that sets forth the purpose of an organization or a component thereof; usually the formation of goals and objectives of the organization or its component.

monitoring and evaluation

A process designed to help organizations effectively use their quality assessment and improvement resources by focusing on high-priority quality-of-care issues. The process includes identification of the most important aspects of care the organization (or department/service) provides; use of indicators to systematically monitor these aspects of care; evaluation of the care at least when thresholds are approached or reached to identify opportunities for improvement or problems; taking action(s) to improve care or solve problems; evaluation of the effectiveness of those actions; and communicating findings through established channels.

nursing staff

Registered nurses, licensed practical/vocational nurses, nursing assistants, and other nursing personnel who perform nursing care in a health care organization.

registered nurse An individual who is qualified by an approved postsecondary program or baccalaureate or higher degree in nursing and is licensed by the state, commonwealth, or territory to practice professional nursing.

organization

The entity through which ambulatory health care services are provided.

organized
Administratively and functionally structured.

outcome
The result(s) of the performance (or nonperformance) of a function or process.

parameters, practice
Strategies for patient management, developed to assist practitioners in clinical decision making. Practice parameters include standards, guidelines, and other patient management strategies.

pathology and medical laboratory services
The services that provide information on diagnosis, prevention, or treatment of disease through the examination of the structural and functional changes in tissues and organs of the body which cause or are caused by disease. Standards are applied to evaluate an organization's performance in providing pathology and medical laboratory services.

> **anatomic pathology** Services relating to surgical pathology, autopsy, and cytology.

> **blood transfusion services** Services relating to transfusing and infusing patients with blood and blood components.

> **clinical pathology** Services relating to the solution of clinical problems, especially the use of laboratory methods in clinical diagnosis; includes clinical chemistry, bacteriology and mycology, parasitology, virology, clinical microscopy, hematology, serology, and radiobioassay.

> **medical technologist, qualified** An individual who is a graduate of a medical technology program approved by a nationally recognized body or who has the documented equivalent in education, training, and/or experience; who meets current legal requirements of licensure or registration; and who is currently competent in the field.

performance
The ability of an individual, group, or organization to carry out those processes that increase the probability of desired outcomes.

> **performance area** An element of the accreditation decision grid consisting of a performance score resulting from aggregation of a number of related standards compliance scores.

> **performance area, key** A performance area that is important in the delivery of quality care.

pharmaceutical services
The activities pertaining to the appropriate, safe, and effective storage, preparation, dispensation, and administration of drugs. Standards are applied to evaluate an organization's performance in providing pharmaceutical services.

> **pharmacist** An individual who has a degree in pharmacy and is licensed and registered to prepare, preserve, compound, and dispense drugs and chemicals.

> **pharmacy** A place where drugs are stored and compounded or dispensed.

physician
An individual who has a degree of doctor of medicine or doctor of osteopathy and who is fully licensed to practice medicine.

plan of correction, conditional accreditation

An organization's written plan, approved by Joint Commission staff, that outlines the activities that the organization will take to address compliance issues that caused the Accreditation Committee to make a decision of conditional accreditation; the plan is the basis for the follow-up survey six months following approval of the plan.

plan of correction, plant, technology, and safety management

An organization's written statement, approved by Joint Commission staff, that details the procedures to be taken to correct existing life safety deficiencies and lists the extraordinary safety measures to be implemented to temporarily reduce the hazards associated with the deficiencies.

plant, technology, and safety management (PTSM)

The organizational management program designed to provide a physical environment free of hazards and to manage staff activities to reduce the risk of human injury. Standards are applied to evaluate an organization's performance in providing plant, technology, and safety management.

podiatrist

An individual who has received the degree of doctor of podiatry medicine and who is licensed to practice podiatry.

policies and procedures

The act, method, or manner of proceeding in some process or course of action or way of doing something, such as policies and procedures governing the medical staff credentialing process.

practice privileges

Permission to render care within well-defined limits based on an individual's professional license and his or her training, experience, competence, ability, and judgment.

process

A goal-directed interrelated series of actions, events, mechanisms, or steps.

> **key process**   A process believed, on the basis of evidence or expert consensus, to increase the probability of desired patient outcome.

program

An outline of work to be done or a prearranged plan of procedure, as in "the program of the administration."

public information interviews

The opportunity during an on-site accreditation survey for the presentation of information by the public or other interested parties, as well as by personnel and staff of the organization undergoing survey.

quality assessment (QA)

The measurement of the technical and interpersonal aspects of health care and service and the outcomes of that care and service. Quality assessment provides information that may be used in quality improvement activities.

quality assessment and improvement

The ongoing activities designed to objectively and systematically evaluate the quality of patient care and services, pursue opportunities to improve patient care and services, and resolve identified problems. Standards are applied to evaluate the quality of an organization's performance in conducting quality assessment and improvement activities.

quality improvement (QI)

An approach to the continuous study and improvement of the processes of providing health care services to meet the needs of patients/residents and others. Synonyms and near-synonyms include continuous quality improvement (CQI), continuous improvement (CI), and total quality management (TQM).

quality of patient care

The degree to which patient care services increase the probability of desired patient outcomes and reduce the probability of undesired outcomes, given the current state of knowledge. Potential components of quality include the following: accessibility of care, appropriateness of care, continuity of care, effectiveness of care, efficacy of care, efficiency of care, patient perspective issues, safety of the care environment, and timeliness of care.

registered nurse

See nursing staff.

respiratory care services

Delivery of care to provide ventilatory support and associated services for patients. Standards are applied to evaluate an organization's performance in providing respiratory care services.

> **respiratory care technician, certified**   An individual who has been certified by the National Board for Respiratory Care after successfully completing all education, experience, and examination requirements.

> **respiratory therapist**   An individual who has successfully completed a training program accredited by the American Medical Association Committee on Allied Health Education and Accreditation in collaboration with the Joint Review Committee for Respiratory Therapy Education and is eligible to take the registry examination administered by the National Board for Respiratory Care, or has the documented equivalent in training and/or experience.

> **respiratory therapy technician**   An individual who has successfully completed a training program accredited by the American Medical Association Committee on Allied Health Education and Accreditation in collaboration with the Joint Review Committee for Respiratory Therapy Education and is eligible to take the certification examination administered by the National Board for Respiratory Care, or has the documented equivalent in training and/or experience.

safety management

A component of an organization's plant, technology, and safety management program that combines five elements—general safety, safety education, emergency preparedness, hazardous materials and waste, and safety devices and operational practices. Standards are applied to evaluate an organization's performance in conducting safety management programs.

scope of care/services

Inventory of processes that make up a specified function including activities performed by governance, managerial, clinical, and/or support personnel.

scoring guideline

See guideline, scoring.

standard

A statement of expectation that defines the structures and processes that must be substantially in place in an organization to enhance the quality of care.

standards manuals   Five Joint Commission books delineating current standards pertaining to specified types of health care organizations. The books are designed for use in organization self-assessment and are the basis for the survey report forms used by the Joint Commission surveyors during on-site surveys. The five manuals are *Accreditation Manual for Hospitals, Accreditation Manual for Long Term Care, Accreditation Manual for Ambulatory Health Care, Accreditation Manual for Home Care,* and *Consolidated Standards Manual.*

summation conference

An optional conference held by surveyors after the chief executive officer exit conference, for all staff and others, designed to convey general observations about the survey findings, and, on the basis of these findings, provide preliminary information about the organization's strengths and weaknesses.

surgical and anesthesia services

Delivery of care for all patients who (1) receive general, spinal, or other major regional anesthesia or (2) undergo surgery or other invasive procedures when receiving general, spinal, or other major regional anesthesia and/or intravenous, intramuscular, or inhalation sedation/analgesia that, in the manner used in the organization, may result in the loss of the patient's protective reflexes. Standards are applied to evaluate an organization's performance in providing surgical and anesthesia services.

survey team

See accreditation survey.

surveyor

See accreditation survey.

tailored survey

See accreditation survey.

threshold

The level or point at which a stimulus is strong enough to signal the need for organization response to indicator data and the beginning of the process of determining why the threshold has been approached or crossed.

type I recommendation

A recommendation or group of recommendations that affect adversely the accreditation decision and should be addressed in the organization's plan for improvement. Progress in resolving type I recommendations is monitored by the Joint Commission through focused surveys, written progress reports, or both at stated times during the accreditation cycle. Failure to resolve such compliance issues within stated time frames can result in the loss of accreditation.

type II recommendation

A recommendation or group of recommendations that are supplementary or consultative in nature and do not affect the accreditation decision. They can, however, affect that decision if not remedied by the time of the next triennial survey.

INDEX

Radiographic services, RS.1.2.1
Radiology services, 45–47
    for emergency services, ES.1.3
    governing body approval of,
        GB.1.3.1.1.9.2
    and medical records, RS.1.4
    policies and procedures, RS.1.7
    space, equipment, and supplies for,
        RS.1.8
    staffing for, RS.1.3, RS.1.5, RS.1.6
Reimbursement, for teaching activities,
        TP.1.1.1
Reports
    administrative, AD.1.1.1.8
    laboratory services and pathology, LP.1.3
    postoperative, SA.1.14, SA.1.15
    quality assessment findings, QA.1.6.2.7.2
    radiology services, RS.1.2.4
    safety management, PL.1.2.4, PL.1.3.1.3,
        PL.1.3.4
Research activities, 57
    adequacy of facilities for, RA.1.4
    appropriateness of, RA.1.3
    monitoring of, RA.1.1.1
    policies and protocol, RA.1, RA.1.1,
        RA.1.2
    rights of subjects, RA.1.5
Risk-assessment program, PL.1.2.2

Safety. *See also* Plant, technology, and safety
        management
    radiology services, RS.1.8.1
    surgical environment, SA.1.21
Safety management. *See* Plant, technology,
        and safety management
Safety officer, PL.1.3
Staffing, GB.1.6
    and emergency preparedness program,
        PL.1.6.3
    in infirmary, IN.1.3, IN.1.4
    for laboratory services and pathology,
        LP.1.4, LP.1.5
    for medical records, MR.1.4
    of pharmaceutical services, PS.1.4

and quality assessment and improvement
        program, QA.1.2
    for radiology services, RS.1.3, RS.1.6
    for safety management program, PL.1.3
    for surgical and anesthesia services,
        SA.1.2, SA.1.3, SA.1.4, SA.1.5,
        SA.1.7, SA.1.8
Sterilized materials, SA.1.21.1.9
Surgical and anesthesia services, 35–40
    anesthesia care coverage, SA.1.13
    and follow-up services, SA.1.19
    history, physical exam, and studies for,
        SA.1.11
    limitations of, SA.1.1
    and medical records, SA.1.14, SA.1.15.1,
        SA.1.16.1, SA.1.17.1.1
    monitoring and evaluation of, QA.1.5.6,
        SA.1.20
    obtaining blood for, SA.1.10
    and patient consent, SA.1.12
    planned, SA.1.1.1
    policies and procedures, SA.1.6
    postoperative discharge, SA.1.17
    and quality of care, SA.1.20
    reports filed after, SA.1.14, SA.1.15
    and resuscitative care, SA.1.18
    safety of environment, SA.1.21
    staffing for, SA.1.2, SA.1.3, SA.1.4,
        SA.1.5, SA.1.7, SA.1.8, SA.1.18
    transfer, SA.1.9

Teaching and publication activities, 55
    policies for publishing, TP.1.3–TP.1.3.3
    reimbursement/compensation for,
        TP.1.1.1
    student/postgraduate training, TP.1.1.3
    supervision of students/trainees, TP.1.2
Test specimens, LP.1.6
Transfers
    of documents/information, QC.1.1.10
    patient, SA.1.9

Utilities management program. *See* Plant,
        technology, and safety management